WELLNESS

to the

CRE

Be Fit, Be Nourished, Be Balanced Beyond *the* Limitations *of* Traditional Medicine

Dr. Jason Sonners, DC, DIBAK, DCBCN, CCWP

RIVER GROVE
BOOKS

Published by River Grove Books
Austin, TX
www.rivergrovebooks.com

Distributed by River Grove Books

For ordering information or special discounts for bulk purchases, please contact River Grove Books at PO Box 91869, Austin, TX 78709, 512.891.6100.

Design and composition by Greenleaf Book Group LLC
Cover design by Greenleaf Book Group LLC
Cover image (apple): ©iStockphoto.com/mixformdesign

Cataloging-in-Publication data
Sonners, Jason.
  Wellness to the core : be fit, be nourished, be balanced beyond the limitations of traditional medicine / Jason Sonners.—1st ed.
    p. : ill. ; cm.
  Issued also as an ebook.
  Includes bibliographical references.
  1. Self-care, Health. 2. Physical fitness. 3. Nutrition. 4. Stress management. 5. Chronic diseases   United States. 6. Well-being. I. Title.
RA776.95 .S66 2014
613   2013951959

Print ISBN: 978-1-938416-60-6
eBook ISBN: 978-1-938416-59-0

First Edition

*This book is dedicated to my children, and to yours.
May it help lead the way to a healthier generation.*

CONTENTS

ACKNOWLEDGMENTS

To Melissa, my wife: Thank you for supporting me as I wrote this book. I could not have completed it without your patience, understanding, and love!

To my children, Levi and Wyatt: Although you are too young to understand this, you are both the driving force for my continued efforts to change the face of health care in this country.

To my family: Thanks to each of you who read the dozens of early drafts of this book. Your thoughts, edits, and comments have all helped to make this book complete.

To Rob Gordon, freelance writer and friend: Without your help, this project may have never gotten off the ground. Your ideas and motivation are greatly appreciated.

To Dr. James Chestnut: I am deeply grateful for the skills, tools, and philosophy you shared with me as your student. You have given me the resources I need to make a positive impact on the people in my life.

INTRODUCTION

It has been well documented that between 75 and 90 percent of chronic illness is the direct result of lifestyle. This means the decisions you make every day regarding your sleep routine, food choices, exercise habits, and how you handle stressful moments directly affect your current level of health. Recognizing the power you have over your health is profound because then you can take responsibility for the way you feel and the way your body functions.

Do you feel good most of the time? Do you wake up feeling refreshed, with plenty of energy to get you through the day? Do you feel totally in control of your stress and daily responsibilities? Do you have loving and supportive relationships with the people who are important to you? Do you actively learn and incorporate new healthy behaviors into your routine? If you answered yes to the above questions, then your doctor would likely find that you have balanced blood sugar, normal cholesterol, normal blood pressure readings, and balanced hormone levels. You would notice that, as time passes, your health improves year after year. If this is true, please continue making the same choices you've been making. You are on the right track!

If, however, you wake up in the morning feeling tired, lacking the energy needed to finish your day, feeling overwhelmed, exhausted, or stressed out, you're feeling warning signs. And, if you are overweight, underappreciated, have high cholesterol or blood pressure, are displeased with your current health, and notice things continue to get worse year after year, it is not too late. You still have the opportunity to change your health.

The first step on the path to wellness is understanding that you *do* have a say in the matter. You are not doomed to be unhealthy, as long as you're willing to do a few things:

- Consider a new approach to your health and your life.
- Make subtle changes to your daily routine.
- Play a proactive role in your health rather than waiting and reacting to each health crisis as it presents itself.

Are you ready to make the commitment to change? Let this book lead your way.

—

Wellness to the Core is divided into two parts. Part One addresses the *causes* of why humans have become so sick. It also clarifies the relationship between our current state of (un)health as a nation and the current health care crisis. Within the parameters of today's "health care" model there is no way out of the cycle of chronic illness and disease that is plaguing our society. Our collective poor health feeds the health care machine and, in turn, the machine facilitates our declining health. It is an exhaustive downward spiral with no real potential to cure or stop the original ailments.

We need a new model—a new way of thinking about health care as a whole that will offer a real solution to the crisis. Part Two offers solutions for getting your health back on track. It outlines the steps you can take to begin the process of reclaiming your health and the life you deserve.

Not everyone reading this book is starting from the same place. Some readers may already be quite healthy and looking for ways to make sure they continue on that track or even to take their health to a higher level. More likely, however, you may be one of the millions of Americans who feel your health slipping away from you. You may even be in a situation that feels hopeless, due to a disease, condition, chronic pain, or predisposition that seems unresolvable. No matter what your current level of health, it is not too late to begin to make changes. As you will see, your health is a continuum on which you are constantly changing your position based on the choices you make. This book can help move you along the health continuum from poor health, through a transitional period, and finally into true health and wellness.

As you read my recommendations, decide where you want to start on your path to wellness. Commit to a few changes. Make those changes part of who you are and then add a few more. You will be improving your health immediately even as you begin to get comfortable with your new routine. As years pass, you will look back and really see that your health has improved instead of deteriorated as you aged.

None of us are as healthy as we can be, and few of us are so sick that we are beyond help. My recommendations apply to the entire population. You may already be doing some of the things I recommend. If so, that's great! Now take it to the next level! Or, you may not be doing any of them yet. That's okay, too. Read through the options and choose changes that you can stick with, that make you happy, and that line up with your goals.

PART ONE

WHY ARE WE SO SICK?

CHAPTER ONE

AMERICA IS IN TROUBLE

—

America is in the throes of a colossal health care crisis. It is evident not only in the increasingly high rates of chronic illness, but also in Americans' inability to deal with, manage, or prevent these widespread diseases. Here are a few facts regarding the health care crisis:

- Almost 50 percent of Americans suffer from a chronic lifestyle disease, such as obesity, high blood pressure, or type 2 diabetes.[1]

- Seven out of ten deaths each year in the US are a result of chronic disease.[2]

- Eighty-seven percent of Americans over sixty-five regularly take prescription drugs.[3]

- Sixty-seven percent of Americans between fifty and sixty-four regularly take prescription drugs.[4]

- The average American takes four prescription drugs on a regular basis.[5]

- Approximately 402 billion prescriptions were written in 2011. That's about fourteen prescriptions for every man, woman, and child in America and that number continues to climb, year after year.

In my health care practice, I talk with hundreds of patients each year from all walks of life. Most of them believe their bodies are breaking down as they get older and there's not much they can do to prevent that deterioration. They believe that a combination of the aging process and bad genes are causing them to be tired, achy, and just plain sick. Most people expect that, as they continue to age, their bodies' ability to regulate normal functions like blood pressure, cholesterol, and hormone balance diminish, and as a result, prescription drugs are required.

Our society looks at the human body like a machine. When the body breaks down, typically as it ages—when it no longer functions the way we think it should—we take it into the shop for repairs. We tend to subscribe to the adage "if it ain't broke don't fix it," especially when it comes to our bodies. Most people wait until they see outward symptoms of sickness before they ask for professional help. But there is a difference between a living organism and a machine. A machine is always going to break down from wear and tear, and parts will need to be replaced over time. But living organisms are not machines. Living organisms have a built-in ability to heal themselves.

Many of my patients are shocked when I tell them that scientific evidence—published in highly respected, peer-reviewed medical journals—clearly shows that our bodies are *not* predestined to break down over time. Scientific evidence shows that the human body is designed for health and balance; your body is constantly trying to return to normal, or "homeostasis," and will do just that if your lifestyle and your environment will allow it to do so.[7]

Many health professionals do not make clear the consequences of living with constant stress, minimal exercise, and unhealthy food. *Premature* breakdown of the human body happens when *something does not allow the body's natural healing to occur*. In other words, when the healing response is equal to the wear and tear, we do not notice any major shifts or deterioration in our body. When the wear and tear exceeds our ability to heal, we notice that things do not feel or function the "way they used to." For most of us, we are finding that our body is not healing as fast or as efficiently as we would like. Overuse, improper use/abuse, or not enough rest and regeneration will slow or stop the healing process. The truth is that modern lifestyles and the environment in which most people live do not promote healing—they promote sickness and disease. Your experience in life and the way you feel will directly reflect the environment you are living in.

In America and throughout the industrialized world, the conventional wisdom about chronic illness is that there is very little we can do about it. Current thinking says:

- Our genes predetermine our health.
- As we age, the diseases we are predetermined to develop gradually kick in.
- Our bodies slowly deteriorate over time, fulfilling our predetermined fate.

The only hope for good health in this scenario is to find out early which diseases we are predetermined to manifest. With that knowledge, we may possibly delay or prevent the damage by taking drugs, removing certain body parts, or even by altering those genes (once science figures out how to do that). Currently, there is evidence that the prevalence of true genetic diseases at birth constitute merely 1 to 2 percent of all the diseases we know of.[8] Clearly this small percentage does not account for all the chronic diseases that are presently being blamed on poor genes.

In recent years, the medical establishment, represented by the American Medical Association (AMA), has begun to accept that a healthy diet and regular exercise may slow down the body's decline. But traditional medicine generally doesn't accept that this decline can be stopped or reversed. Moreover, it does not give appropriate weight to the impact that lifestyle and environment play in our health. The gene control belief system—that is, conventional wisdom—is, more than any other single factor, what holds people helpless and hopeless in the deterioration of their physical bodies. But this is not the truth. Your body wants to be healthy! You might be asking, "If my genes do not determine my level of health, what does?" It's simple: Your choices do.

In almost all cases, your health is determined foremost by the quality of your choices regarding the foods you eat, the way you treat and move your body, and the way you approach and view your life, including your belief system, attitudes, self-esteem, and stress management skills. Some people think that eating healthy means depriving themselves. Choosing health does not mean deprivation! You might see deprivation as giving up sweets or cutting back on caffeine. That is not *real* deprivation. Deprivation is allowing your body and mind to deteriorate to the point where you cannot enjoy your life, enjoy time with your family, or contribute to your community. Being deprived is allowing yourself to get so sick or so weak that you lose your independence and continue life without satisfaction or fulfillment.

⁓

In the past twenty years, the average American life span has increased from sixty-five to seventy-seven years, and it's still increasing.[9] In fact, many of us will live to the ages of eighty, ninety, or even one hundred. Some of the reasons for increasing longevity are major advances in medicine and hygiene. Before chronic diseases became the epidemic they are today, the leading causes of death were infection and life-threatening trauma. Cleaner living conditions, antibiotics to treat severe infection, and medical treatments for trauma have contributed significantly to increasing longevity.

Yet, we have all noticed that some people in their seventies, eighties, and nineties appear to be much older and their quality of life seems very low. Seeing them, you may think, "I don't want to look and feel the way they do." Although life expectancy has increased to seventy-seven, the quality of life index remains at about that of a sixty-year-old.[10] So, while Americans are living longer, their quality of life tends to decrease dramatically after age sixty. The difference between you and today's eighty- and ninety-year-olds is that, when they were young, they had no idea that they were going to live so long. They also had no idea that the choices they made in their twenties, thirties, forties, fifties, and sixties would make them look and feel so badly in their seventies, eighties, and nineties. You do now! So, the real question is not, "Will I live to a ripe old age?" You likely will! The question you should ask is, "What is my quality of life going to be when I get there?"

It all comes down to choices, and your choices stem from your beliefs. If your health is valuable to you and you believe that exercise is a necessary part of being healthy, then the likelihood of you exercising is pretty high. If you believe that you do not have time to exercise or you believe that you do not like to exercise, then the likelihood of you participating in exercise is very low. Whether you realize it or not, your beliefs about your life, your health, what you deserve, and what you value are determining your choices all the time.

Most of us do not realize the impact good choices have on our lives. We make choices based on whatever we want in the moment. If you decide to follow a particular behavior or eat a certain food, it usually has to do with what you want or what you decide is important. Often we don't see past immediate gratification to realize the consequences of our choices, nor do we evaluate the risk-benefit analysis for our choices.

Health doesn't have to be about choosing *not* to eat cookies and brownies by the bagful or choosing *not* to sit on the couch watching television. I know this appears to be depriving behavior. But, if you just switch around your thoughts, it can be about choosing a healthy diet, choosing to move your body—making choices that make you healthier. Although you may feel that reducing your consumption of brownies, ice cream, and TV time is depriving yourself of pleasure, indulging too much is what is really depriving you of good health. When you change your mindset and reorient your beliefs, you are actually *choosing* health.

When you make steps to improve your lifestyle, the potential outcome of improved health happens regardless of whether it "feels" good or it "feels" like deprivation. The difference is that when it feels good, your chances of sticking to it are much higher, thus maximizing your opportunity for success. Remember, the choices you make today *will* absolutely affect your health in the future. Hundreds of my patients have opened up to this way of thinking. They have learned that making healthy choices brings with it the signs of improved health, such as better digestion, more energy, positive emotions, more fun, and more free time to spend doing things they enjoy. Does that sound like deprivation to you?

Do you think it's possible that your health can improve over the next five years? I hope your answer is an enthusiastic "Yes!"

CASE STUDY: YOUR BODY RESPONDS TO THE ENVIRONMENT IN WHICH IT DWELLS.

Brian, a sixty-three-year-old male patient, came to me with recurring lower-back stiffness, which felt especially bad when he first woke up. Although the stiffness seemed to work itself out during the day, it never fully resolved. Then, sure enough, it was back again the next morning.

Brian commented during his first visit that one of the questions on the initial intake form asked if he planned on being healthier five years from now. He laughed and said, "Don't you think it's a little too late for me?"

I responded, "Absolutely not! Why would it be?" I'm not sure he believed me at that particular moment, but he did follow through with my recommendations, including making dietary changes, taking supplements, and following an exercise and stretching routine. Now, four years later, Brian often mentions that first visit and his surprise that, at sixty-seven years old, he feels better than he did ten or fifteen years ago.

Brian, like many Americans, was under the assumption that as we age we should expect to get sicker, have more aches and pains, and accept these losses in quality of life as just part of the "normal" aging process. Now, as a result of going through our programs, Brian knows firsthand that this does not need to be the case.

CHAPTER TWO

THE PARADIGM PROBLEM

—

At the core of our society's health crisis is the current "health care" paradigm—our accepted model or pattern for health and "health care." More and more, it's apparent that the way we have been viewing health and physiology has been inaccurate. But that is changing as we learn that the beliefs we collectively held about health and health care aren't necessarily true.

Since the early twenty-first century, the prevailing understanding of human health and physiology has been driven by the "Central Dogma," a theory developed by Francis Crick, one part of the team of scientists who discovered DNA. Crick's Central Dogma states, "Genes control our biology and physiology, and therefore our health is predetermined by these genes." According to this theory, health would be predetermined at birth and we would be helpless to try to become healthier than our genes allow. Perhaps this is why scientists continue to invest so much time and money searching for the genes associated with obesity, cancer, diabetes, and other common conditions. The Central Dogma, or gene control theory, taught to our young doctors does not reflect the full story. And yet, despite its lack of completeness, this fundamental principle is not only considered an unassailable truth; it is revered in the medical world.

Following the Central Dogma there would be only one answer to the most important question I ask my patients: "Is it possible that your health could be better five years from now?" The answer would always be, "No!"

According to gene theory, if we have "bad genes," all we can do is delay the inevitable biological breakdown. If we're lucky, we might be able to make our unavoidable, preordained, disease-ridden, slow-but-inevitable decline a bit less painful. But that's all we can hope for, because our genetic code dooms us to spend our "golden years" in dysfunction and disease, limited in our activities, confined to a nursing home, or worse.

Does this sound familiar? It probably does, because this is what most people have heard throughout their lives. The medical world takes gene theory very seriously and, as a result, doctors spend huge amounts of time and pharmaceutical companies spend huge amounts of money identifying and trying to "fix" or alter genes. They believe that altering the "bad" genes will change the way they function in our bodies. Rather than curing or preventing diseases like cancer and diabetes, they are just increasing our life expectancy after the problems manifest.

The problem with the Central Dogma and gene control theory is that while it is absolutely true that genes dictate our physiology, there is more to the story. Genes only contain instructions; in fact, they contain all of the instructions necessary for biological life, but they have no ability to decide the best response. This means that genes wait for cues from the environment and respond accordingly. For example, there might be a "type 2 diabetes gene" responsible for how the body tolerates sugar. Everyone would carry the gene, but some people may have a stronger tolerance for sugars than others. Therefore some people may be predisposed to develop diabetes when compared to people with a higher tolerance. While predispositions may exist, a person would still need to be exposed to high levels of sugar, processed grains and corn, high stress, and a sedentary lifestyle in order for the gene to manifest type 2 diabetes. If that same person refrained from a high-sugar, high-stress lifestyle, it would not matter that the predisposition for diabetes existed. The gene would not be able to express itself without the environmental cue.

Unlike the "gene control" theory, supporting evidence for the theory that genes require environmental cues is very strong and can be found in numerous carefully controlled medical research studies.[11] An entire scientific discipline called epigenetics has emerged to study the fact that our environment ultimately controls our genes. Yet, because the Central Dogma is such an accepted part of the medical worldview, epigenetics remains largely ignored.

It is neither controversial nor inaccurate to say that we are getting sicker and sicker every year. It is well documented that the overall health in industrialized nations (including the US) is declining rapidly. Meanwhile, doctors continue trying to address and alter genes because their paradigm holds that it is genes that cause disease. But, we must dig deeper and ask, Why are our genes behaving this way? Are we legitimately designed for sickness or are we designed for health? If genes have no autonomy for decision making, then genes cannot be the catalyst for what they do. They are simply doing exactly what they are supposed to: responding to environmental signals. Here's how it works: Genes instruct your body to respond to environmental cues. Without a signal from the environment, there is no response. It follows that positive input creates a positive response, and negative input creates a negative response.

Medical microbiologist Bruce Lipton, PhD, performed an experiment that demonstrated this point very well. You might recall from high school biology that the nucleus of a cell is called its "brain" because it contains all the cell's genes and is its control center. We all know what would happen if we separated the brain from the body, but until Lipton's experiment, we did not know what would happen when the nucleus was removed from the cell.

Want to take a guess what happened when Lipton removed the nucleus from human cells? The cells not only continued to live, but they continued to eat, digest, and avoid toxins.[12] Some cells lived as long as a few months, disproving our belief that this was simply impossible. Dr. Lipton's experiment proved that cell "brains" (DNA) do not, in fact, control cell function. It was a small step, then, for him to conclude that genes do not control life function. Based on this research, Dr. Lipton and other epigenetic scientists estimate that between 75 and 90 percent (or more) of the current chronic diseases are not caused by genes alone.[13]

You're probably thinking, "Wow! What a breakthrough. Great news!" But is it? Dr. Lipton's discovery is good or bad depending on your point of view. It shows that we are *not* helpless as we try to maintain or improve our health. That's certainly good news. But it also means that we are responsible—very much responsible—for both our health *and* our illness.

Here's a great analogy by Dr. James Chestnut, chiropractor, lecturer, and educator: Imagine you're a biologist studying a lake and its surrounding ecosystem. Suddenly, without warning or visible cause, the lake population begins dying at a rapid rate. You gather some of the dead and dying fish, and as you study them, you find that they are suffering from rare diseases. What would be your initial thought as to why they were dying? Would you think that, somehow, a rapid genetic mutation was occurring? Or, would you think that something in the water (i.e. the environment) was causing the fish to die? It would likely be the latter hypothesis, according to Dr. Chestnut's analogy, because the environment directly impacts the health of our genes and thus, our bodies.

Now that we are becoming more chronically ill, should we assume that our genes have suddenly mutated? I don't think so. It's inarguable that a rapid increase in previously rare chronic diseases is plaguing our society, and rates of heart disease, cancer, stroke, and diabetes are skyrocketing every year.[14] It is also inarguable that human genes have been basically unchanged for the past forty thousand years.[15] Therefore, it seems to follow that the only factors changing as rapidly as our declining health are the choices we are making and the environment in which we live.

CASE STUDY: THE PARADIGM PROBLEM IN A NUTSHELL.

Stacy, a twenty-one-year-old female, complained of irritable bowel syndrome (IBS). She had already seen three different gastrointestinal specialists but felt no relief from her symptoms. Her mother, who was already a patient of mine, encouraged her to see me. I asked Stacy to bring any previous test results, blood work, and colonoscopy or endoscopy results from her previous doctor visits.

We discussed her diet, which was heavy in carbohydrates like wheat, sugar, and other grains. We discussed her blood work results, which indicated gluten intolerance. When I inquired about her test results, she told me that her previous doctors told her not to worry because her "IBS was not food related."

I told Stacy I couldn't imagine why any doctor would say that, as the tests clearly indicated sensitivity to gluten (the protein found in wheat and other grains). I explained that it was very possible that eating gluten on a regular basis was creating an unhealthy environment within her stomach and intestines, producing inflammation, gas, bloating, and indigestion. Before we proceeded with additional treatments, I asked her to eliminate gluten from her diet to confirm that it was the main contributor to her problem. When I asked her if that was something she was willing to do, she said, "Yes, I have no problem with that; I just haven't done that yet because the other doctors told me not to. They told me my problem was related to having too much stress in my life."

I have yet to meet a patient with non-food-related IBS. In

Stacy's case, at least one of the definite irritants was gluten. Within three to four weeks of removing gluten and adding a few digestive enzymes to help her body digest other foods, Stacy was perfectly fine. The chronic inflammation and irritation associated with this environment (her body) had never allowed her intestines to heal from the irritation. Once we determined the cause of the inflammation and removed it from her intestines, her body could clean up that environment and allow her intestines to heal.

Ironically, while studying to become a physician assistant (PA), Stacy presented her own case study to her professor, an MD. He told her that most likely her gluten intolerance was all in her head, that based on her tests, she was not allergic to gluten and her successful recovery was psychosomatic; it worked because she believed it would, not because of how she adjusted her diet to resolve the problem. As a result of the professor's disbelief in the IBS case study, he selected someone else to lead the workshop instead of Stacy.

What a perfect example of how the traditional medical paradigm fails people. My heart immediately sank for Stacy. Here was a young woman with a major personal success story regarding her health, excited to share it with her class, only to be disappointed and embarrassed by her professor because he could only view her disease through his conventional paradigm. He could not see the transitional levels of health—the gray area between dysfunction and disease. He could not see nor would he look for the subtle changes exhibited by the body, nor did he believe that intestinal problems could be caused by the food a person eats. This is a tragedy and a failing of our medical system.

CHAPTER THREE

WHY IS YOUR
HEALTH DECLINING?

At this moment in history, humans as a whole are very sick. Have you ever heard of another species experiencing the levels of chronic lifestyle diseases that we have? Do you ever hear of epidemic levels of heart disease or cancer in elephants or alligators? That may sound ridiculous to you, but humans are animals, too. So why do we have such high incidences of these diseases? The only other animals that show high levels of these diseases are our cats and dogs. This is most likely because they share in our lifestyle.

Humans around the world are sick, but Americans are *really* sick:

- The number of prescription drugs per person DOUBLES every decade.[16]

- The amount of money spent on prescription drugs DOUBLES every decade.[17]

- Americans make up 5 percent of the world's population, and we use 50 percent of the world's health care dollars.[18]

- The United States spends $1.6 trillion on health care each year. This is four times the amount spent on defense and forty times the amount spent on homeland security.[19]

- Today, 76 percent (more than three-quarters) of Americans regularly take prescription drugs.[20]

Yet with all this research and spending:

- Today, 46 percent (that's almost half) of Americans are suffering from a chronic lifestyle disease like diabetes or heart disease.[21]
- Heart disease is expected to double in the next fifty years.[22]
- Sixty percent of America is overweight.[23]
- Rates of obesity have gone up 50 percent in the past ten years.[24]
- We are currently ranked as the thirty-seventh healthiest country.[25]

Wouldn't you expect more from a world leader?

We spend more money, conduct more research, take more drugs, remove and replace more body parts, and yet we're getting sicker and sicker each year. Worse still, there doesn't appear to be a solution available in our current system. Here's a snapshot of how much money the United States spends on chronic disease:

- $500 million on heart disease (America's number-one killer)[26]
- $430 million on cancer (the number-two killer)[27]
- $670 million on diabetes[28]
- $402 million on obesity[29]
- $337 million on digestive disorders[30]
- $220 million on arthritis[31]
- $38 million on the fractures related only to osteoporosis[32]

Do those numbers seem big to you? They're large sums, all right, but they're actually bigger than you think: Those are the total dollars spent in America, not per year, not per month, but *every single day.*

And that's not all. Every day, we spend more than $46 million on the research, development, and marketing of new drugs.[33] In fact, our prescription drug spending has doubled in the past ten years.[34] Is this spending for the creation of drugs that will prevent diseases or change our body structure to make us immune to diseases? Neither. The vast majority of that money is being poured into finding ways to ease symptoms, thus keeping us alive but still diseased. There is very little, if any, effort put into looking for the underlying cause of disease or attempting to prevent diseases from occurring in the first place. In the face of these facts, trying to get healthy and improve your life can seem like an insurmountable challenge.

As if that's not enough, consider this: More than four hundred thousand people die every year from medical intervention, such as surgeries gone wrong, hospital-borne infections, and drug interactions. The American Medical Association has acknowledged that modern medicine is the third leading cause of death in the United States. This may even be a conservative estimate. An article in *Life Extension* magazine entitled "Death by Medicine" states that medical interventions are the number one cause of death in the United States—*the number one cause.*[35]

Our health care system is charged with the responsibility to improve our health and cure disease. Instead, our population's health declines year after year. We find that we are prescribed more medications but keep developing new symptoms and syndromes. This system is making us dependent on medical therapies to manage symptoms rather than teaching us what we can do to improve our health. This lack of education is creating a victim mindset among our population. It has created a lack of concern and lack of interest in trying to take care of ourselves and to properly prevent these diseases. As a result we do not experience life the way we were designed to—as healthy, happy, active, unrestricted, pain-free members of our community. Is this a system we can trust with our health, or should we be looking for a better path toward improved health?

While we do not rate very high on the list of healthiest countries, we do excel at trauma care and emergency medicine. With accidents, injuries, or when our bodies are too far gone for anything else to work, surgery and medication can and must play a vital role. But, it's more important to do anything and everything to be and remain as healthy as we can for as long as we can. If we do that, the mainstream health care system becomes an option of last resort, to be used only when absolutely necessary.

The good news is there is a viable, effective alternative to traditional medicine to play the role in prevention and maintenance of our health. Holistic medicine focuses on keeping you as healthy and balanced as possible. It looks at you and your life as a whole and helps you be more proactive with your health rather than waiting until you are sick before stepping in. The key is to use holistic health care to keep your *whole* body as healthy as possible for as long as possible, and to visit traditional medical doctors when things go awry.

Modern medicine has its place, and it's an important place. I don't believe that holistic medicine could or should replace modern medicine, mostly because each one deals with different types of problems. Holistic medicine must work in tandem with modern medicine for the overall benefit of you, the patient! We need to educate the public on the causes of illness and what they should do to get well and stay well. We're all going to need to learn more about our health and how to maintain it. Then, people will use this knowledge to help them make healthier decisions.

⌣

The intake form we use for new patients in our office is a good snapshot of my holistic approach to health and wellness, and I've been told that it's pretty unusual. Four key questions from the form are:

- How long has it been since you really felt good?
- Are you healthier today than you were five years ago?
- Do you plan on being healthier five years from now?
- If so, how do you plan to make that happen?

Why do we ask these questions? It's simple. Remember, your body *wants* to be healthy. Because your body prefers health and is always trying to get healthy, there is no reason why you can't be healthier five years from now than you are today. All you need is a plan that will lead you toward better health, one step at a time.

Like all living things, our bodies are designed for good health. It actually takes a lot of time and abuse to make a human body chronically ill. Yet, many people won't start to feel poorly until thirty or forty years of age. It's fascinating to me when people say: "Doc, I don't know why I feel so bad. I'm not doing anything different now than I've ever done. I mean, I've been living this way my whole life! Why now, all of a sudden, am I being affected this way?" Then they tell me how they've been living and describe the kind of abuse they've been putting themselves through for years and years. I hear how they've been working long hours under near-constant stress. They tell me they skip breakfast or eat something sugary, grab something greasy and starchy for lunch, and maybe also for dinner. If they get any exercise at all, it's only on the weekend, and then they typically overdo it. Then they are sedentary the remaining hours of the day and rarely get enough sleep.

So why now, all of a sudden, are they being affected negatively? It's because they have been living this way for many years and the unhealthy lifestyle is starting to catch up with them. Our miraculous bodies work very hard to protect us from deficiencies in vitamins and minerals. They strive daily to overcome the toxins in our environment. They do everything they can, and they wait for us to change our ways. But many people never change. Finally, exhausted, the body gives up the fight and starts to show signs of chronic disease.

The most impressive fact to me is that our bodies can actually withstand all that neglect for thirty or forty years before exhibiting any sign of diseases. Of course, physical decline is accelerating, as we can now see our children beginning to show signs of chronic disease as early as nine or ten years old.

~

There are pros and cons to almost all decisions we make. As people experience the positive benefits of making healthy decisions, they become much more willing and able to stay on a path that promotes health and healing rather than one that robs them of their health and quality of life.

At any point, you can learn how to create the appropriate environment within your own life and body to promote health and healing. I call it the **Be Fit, Be Nourished, Be Balanced** program, and you'll learn more about it in Part Two. The approach will be slightly different for each person—there is no singular solution to everyone's health issues. But if you carefully follow the program, you will begin to see and feel improvements and then continue to improve until you reach the optimum health for your age and personal situation. However, if you stop your program and are no longer taking care of yourself, you will also stop improving and, eventually, lose the progress you have made.

CASE STUDY: YOU CAN ONLY COMPENSATE FOR SO LONG BEFORE THE BODY GIVES UP.

Chris, a thirty-nine-year-old male, visited my practice to see if we could help with his allergies. His initial complaints were typical symptoms like sinus congestion, watery eyes, itchy throat, and constant post-nasal drip. He told us that he had these issues year round. The symptoms had started two years earlier, and before that he had never suffered from any allergies.

His primary care physician put him on allergy medication (which doesn't cure the allergies but should help relieve the symptoms) and told him a person can grow out of or develop allergies at any age and that there is really no rhyme or reason as to why this happens. Chris then saw an ear, nose, and throat doctor (ENT) who said he might recommend surgery to help widen the sinus cavity to allow for better drainage. Not wanting to be on allergy medication and trying to avoid surgery, he came to us hoping for an alternative.

With a busy sales job, Chris left the house very early each day to get on the road; most days he had appointments all day and did not get home until fairly late in the evening. Most mornings he had just a cup of coffee for breakfast (with cream and sugar), and he often grabbed fast food for lunch. If he made it home for dinner he would eat a pretty healthy balanced meal that his wife would prepare, but if he wasn't home for dinner, he might eat fast food again or pizza. Chris also admitted to having a pretty big sweet tooth and loved to snack on candy between meals. He described his schedule as demanding but denied feeling overwhelmed or overstressed. He had been working and living this way for almost twenty years.

I explained to Chris that allergies are an overreaction of the immune system to some outside irritant. His condition did not seem to be seasonal in nature, as he indicated he felt this way year round. So he must have been allergic to something he was in contact with year round. I was concerned that his work schedule and his diet were very unhealthy; plus, he spent his day sitting in his car or in meetings, not getting much movement. I told him that in addition to his allergies, his lifestyle would likely lead to other health issues down the road.

I put him on a plan, focusing first on his sugar intake. Sugar suppresses immune function significantly. I had him take the milk and sugar out of his coffee, and we traded candy snacks for trail mix, apples, and berries. I also had him eat a hard-boiled egg every morning for breakfast to help stabilize his morning blood sugar. With those changes alone, in two-and-a-half weeks his allergy symptoms improved by half. This motivated him to want more results. From there we continued to modify his diet by finding healthy options for his lunches on-the-go and making a commitment to get home for a healthy dinner. I also got him to commit to exercising for at least one hour every Saturday and Sunday. It took another three months, but his allergy symptoms continued to reduce. Because allergies are an overreaction to an environmental stimuli (pollen, mold, foods, dust, etc.), it takes time to build the immune system back up to a level strong enough to tolerate these factors. With Chris's lifestyle changes, he successfully reversed his condition.

CHAPTER FOUR

STRESS

In chiropractic medicine, the field in which I was trained, it is well accepted that health comes from the inside out, not from the outside in. But, health *problems* often do come from the outside in—in the form of stress.

Like all living things, human bodies are self-regulating and self-healing. For example, when your body gets cold, it recognizes a change and raises your core temperature by shivering. When you eat, your body knows that it has to digest the food to get nutrients. If you get injured, your body immediately begins to heal the wound. Similarly, your body has a built-in and very logical response when it is trying to cope with various kinds of stress.

Stress is a multidimensional and complex force, either positive or negative, that causes us to change in some way. It is also a personal experience, meaning that not all people will respond to the same stressors the same way. Positive, healthy stress is called *eustress*, while negative or unhealthy stress is called *distress*. Distress will always push you toward sickness and away from health. There are three primary sources of stress:

- **Physical stress** (what you do to your body) includes injuries but can also include minor physical irritations caused by common daily activities like manual labor, repetitive motions, an active lifestyle, work around the home or in the yard, or even sitting at a desk or sleeping on a bad mattress.

- **Chemical stress** (what you put in your body) includes drugs, alcohol, cigarettes, vitamins, water, and food.
- **Emotional stress** (what you think about) is caused by negative thoughts or feelings, including worry, anxiety, neurosis, mental illness, anger, resentment, frustration, or a sense of powerlessness.

Causes of distress can include poor food choices, sedentary living, or mourning a death in the family. Eustress is "healthy" stress. While it does stress your body and mind, eustress has a positive overall impact that moves you away from sickness and toward health. Examples of eustress may include digesting a balanced breakfast, getting proper exercise, and the birth of a baby. Although exercise is physically *stressful*, getting the proper amount and type of exercise would be considered eustress.

Stress has always been a component of human life, but in today's world, it has become one of the major causes of disease. So, learning how to better manage stress and creating a balance of eustress and distress is paramount for health and healing. In fact, while stress has become a major cause for the human body to get so ill, balancing your distress and your eustress will give your body the opportunity to do what it does so well: heal.

Stress is the greatest lifestyle problem Americans face today. And the only way to fix a problem caused by lifestyle is to alter that lifestyle. Think of your health as a math equation:

$$\frac{\textbf{WHAT YOU DO FOR YOUR BODY} - \textbf{WHAT YOU DO TO YOUR BODY}}{\textbf{YOUR CURRENT LEVEL OF HEALTH}}$$

The important thing is to find ways to balance the equation of your life. If you can do that, you will help your body to balance itself, too.

I'll make you a promise: If you can make a few positive life-style changes, like beginning to control stress and adopting a program designed to put you on the path to wellness, your health will dramatically improve, and it can start improving immediately. It really doesn't matter where your health is today; you can change it. If you are willing to make positive lifestyle changes, you will likely become the healthiest you have been in years. What's more, there is absolutely no reason why you cannot continue that positive health trend for years to come.

CASE STUDY: WE ALL EXPERIENCE STRESS DIFFERENTLY.

Eric, a fifteen-year-old male, had "the feeling of having the flu every day": a history of fatigue, dizziness, constipation, an unwillingness to get out of bed each morning, and all-over achiness.

Diagnosed with fibromyalgia, he had recently been put on an antidepressant. He was also prescribed various drugs for his fatigue and dizziness. He explained that his high school advanced-placement classes were very stressful, and he felt overwhelmed with the amount of work expected of him. He had even quit playing sports due to his lack of energy and feeling faint on the field.

I addressed Eric's lifestyle issues, getting him into healthy sleep patterns and altering his diet from various angles. Not only was his diet deficient in important nutrients, it was filled with processed foods, pesticides, artificial sweeteners, and inflammatory chemicals. It's amazing to me that we do not often consider things like food and lifestyle with these symptoms. Food is our fuel. If we are not getting the proper fuel in our body, how can we expect it to perform properly?

After a few weeks we introduced a slow full-body exercise program to get him moving again. Gradually, over the next few months, Eric began to experience what being a teenager was supposed to feel like. He is now in college and playing intramural sports with plenty of energy to sustain him.

You can see how the three sources of negative stress (physical, chemical, and emotional) affected Eric. Due to their conventional medical paradigm, his medical doctors did not have a way to understand his situation nor the tools to help him. If you cannot test for and diagnose a problem, then you do not see it or think it exists. You cannot cure, fix, or effectively manage a problem without a proper set of tools. Lifestyle conditions require lifestyle remedies, not drugs or surgery.

CHAPTER FIVE

THE STRESS RESPONSE

—

If distress is one of the key reasons for poor health, then effectively dealing with distress is a key way to improve health—because the only way to really solve a problem is to address the cause of that problem. It is impossible to solve a problem by simply removing the symptoms, which is the way that prescription drugs often work. While that may buy you some time, you must take care of the underlying causes if you want a real, lasting solution.

If you are exposed to distress, big or small, acute or chronic, your body produces the "stress response." Understanding the stress response will help you see what is causing the kinds of illnesses that are so prevalent today.

Here is what happens to your body when it is under stress:[36]

- Increased heart rate
- Blood vessel constriction, leading to increased blood pressure
- Increased LDL (bad) cholesterol
- Decreased HDL (good) cholesterol
- Decreased immune response
- Decreased short-term memory
- Decreased capacity for learning

- Increased insulin resistance
- Increased blood glucose levels
- Increased blood clotting factors

This list comprises the body's short-term biological reaction—the "flight or fight" response—that is its very sensible way of dealing with an immediate threat. The fight or flight response prepares you to either run away from danger or fight off the enemy. Human bodies were designed to handle stress very effectively, but only for short periods of time. If the stress response occurs in your body too often or for too long, the changes that are helpful in the short term can lead to major health problems in the long term, such as chronic conditions like high blood pressure, diabetes, cancer, cholesterol imbalances, heart disease, ADD/ADHD, dementia, stroke, and many more.

Modern life is filled to the brim with conditions that keep you in a state of almost continuous stress. You wake up in the morning and rush to get ready for work. You eat unhealthy food for breakfast—if you eat at all. When you eat healthy food, you often eat it too fast. You drive to work on crowded roads surrounded by drivers who frustrate you. You arrive at work only to feel overwhelmed by your workload and deadlines. Day after day, life seems to go on this way.

The important thing to know is that the stress response is a perfectly normal reaction and is not designed to make you sick—unless you overdo it. It is not pathology (illness); it does not need drugs to keep it under control. What is needed is an understanding of what is happening inside so you can take steps to correct these imbalances. The difference between stress today and the stress people typically experienced 150 years ago is that today's stress is now constant and at a high level. There is little or no time for recovery and healing. When was the last time you took a real vacation? How about a vacation without phones, email, text messages, or the Internet?

When you live in conditions of chronic stress, your body is in a state of catabolism, *breaking you down* rather than *healing you*. Why? Your body literally breaks itself down to provide you with the raw materials needed for survival in hopes the stress will go away and you can return to a state of healing and recovery. It does this to save your life. The human body can only keep the stress response up for so long before it starts to wear you down. So its responses are *not* signs of illness; they are normal and appropriate changes in response to chronic stress. The environment you are in and your lifestyle is the problem—not your body. If you are under constant stress at work or at home—or both—and you start feeling overwhelmed or sick, it's not that your body is ill; it's that you're in a terribly stressful situation. You need to change the environment.

It follows that if there are three sources of stress (physical, emotional, and chemical) that impact your health, then healing must occur on all three fronts as well. To demonstrate how the feedback loop works, consider emotional eating. Perhaps, when you're distressed or sad, you reach for a comforting food like ice cream or chips. Rather than having one scoop or a handful of chips, you eat the whole container. Not only has your emotional state led to overeating, you might also end up with an upset stomach from consuming too much unhealthy food. And then you're right back where you started: feeling sick, likely still stressed out, and maybe even upset that you've blown your healthy eating habit. All three stressors affect the other components of stress collectively and cumulatively. But you can use that interrelationship to your advantage—to heal yourself. You can exercise to feel better emotionally and physically. You can reduce emotional stress and improve the way you digest your food. You can eat healthier to feel better physically and/or emotionally. And so the cycle continues, but as a positive feedback loop.

To be healthy, you'll need to take a dynamic approach to stress. You'll need to find which stressors are causing the problems and then develop a plan for decreasing the negative effects on your body and mind. Your plan must involve the food you eat, the way you move your body, and the way you approach your life emotionally.

CASE STUDY: STRESS AFFECTS EACH PERSON DIFFERENTLY.

Cynthia originally came to our office for "wellness" adjustments. This means she did not have any glaring issue that she wanted resolved—no pain, no headaches—she just wanted her body "tuned up" periodically. Cynthia was new to the area. She had relocated to New Jersey for a new job. She had found that getting regular adjustments helped keep her body less stressed. We approached her treatments from this philosophy for many months.

As time went on, I noticed that she, like many other people, held her tension in her neck and shoulders. When she had a particularly stressful week I could feel the tightness build in her shoulders. The adjustments we had been making were effective in reducing her muscle tension and providing her with relief but her stress would build up agian rather quickly. She would tell me that her new job was more stressful and demanding than her previous position.

After about a year, she began having an increase in joint pain. The joint pain seemed to move around. Sometimes it would show up in her elbows, her back, or even in her hips and knees. She spent a great deal of time hiking and camping, so I first recommended she get tested for Lyme disease. She went to her primary doctor and they ran extensive Lyme panels and rheumatoid factors, which showed absolutely nothing. Our next step was to discuss diet and lifestyle.

She, like so many other Americans, ate an inflammatory diet filled with fast foods, processed foods, and diet beverages. We discussed the effect these foods could be having on her body when she disagreed, telling me, "I've been eating this way for fifteen or twenty years. Why would this be happening to me now?" I explained to her that this may have always been an issue for her, but for years her body was compensating and clearing out those toxins fast enough to avoid any symptoms from the chemicals in the processed food. Perhaps now, years later and with the increased demands at work, that total amount of stress on her was too much and her body was no longer able to tolerate these foods.

We made some simple adjustments to her diet as well as kept up with regular adjustments. It took about nine weeks, but her joint pain slowly diminished until it was completely gone. Cynthia does still get an occasional flare-up of the joint pain, but it always coincides with a time she strays from her new way of eating.

The cumulative effects of stress are different for everyone. Stress can affect any of the body's functional systems. For some people it shows up as muscle tension in the neck, back, or jaw; for others it can be allergy symptoms, digestive issues, joint pain, blood sugar imbalances, brain fog, fatigue, a short temper, or any number of other issues. The important thing to understand is that these symptoms are not normal. They are your body's way of telling you something must change. Almost every time, that "something" is the way you treat your body. If you want to keep your body running properly you must take the best care of it that you can. Your lifestyle, in the long run, has the biggest impact on your health—more so than anything else.

CHAPTER SIX

ENVIRONMENT, LIFESTYLE, AND YOUR HEALTH

~

Anthropologists and zoologists have a good system for determining the right environment for a given animal. It's quite revolutionary, really—they watch the animal in its natural habitat. By doing this, they get a feel for what its natural diet should be, how the animals naturally interact with one another socially, and what their typical energy expenditure is.

When animals live in their natural environments, they thrive. They experience almost no chronic lifestyle disease. When we alter their environment—like domesticating them, feeding them processed foods, or placing them in confined or unnatural habitats, they begin to experience increased illness. Aren't humans animals, too? Yes. But does our current environment reflect what is natural and good for us? Absolutely not![37]

In the course of only one or two centuries, we have changed our environment so drastically we don't even know what an ideal human environment looks like. We live sedentary lives oriented around our couches and desk chairs. We eat significantly more processed foods than real, whole foods. We are exposed to hundreds if not thousands of man-made chemicals in our air, food, and water supplies. We no longer live in tight-knit, supportive communities. Having altered our natural habitat so dramatically, we are literally making ourselves sick and dying from our decisions and lifestyles. What can we do about that? Can we just give up on modern civilization and return to life in the jungle, the mountains, or the desert?

When we study hunter-gatherer civilizations, whether past or present, we see certain differences compared with modern lifestyles. For instance, hunters and gatherers moved their bodies all day. Whether they were hunting or gathering, working or playing, they were very active all the time. Their diets were also much different from ours. They ate only fruits, vegetables, nuts, seeds, and meat. No chips, cake, or candy; not even bread. Certainly they ate no processed, calorie-dense foods devoid of nutrients, or chemically or genetically altered foods. Is it surprising that they didn't experience lifestyle-related chronic illness like we do? Not at all.

As an example, let's take the Native American populations. It's well documented that Native Americans have a high incidence of diabetes. Why? Most medical scientists seem to believe that diabetes is genetic within that population. The issue, however, is not their genes; it's exposing their genes to an unnatural diet containing foods they were not genetically designed to consume and that adversely affect their health. Just a few hundred years ago, diabetes was rare in Native American families, with almost no incidence at all. It wasn't until they adopted a sedentary lifestyle and began eating a Western diet that the disease became a "genetic" epidemic.[38]

We should at least acknowledge that, just as there is a natural environment for grizzly bears and gorillas, there is a natural environment for humans. There is an environment where we can thrive and achieve our natural level of health. Within that environment, there are natural human behaviors that promote healthy living.

Our ancestors lived in that environment, and they thrived.[39] There are places on the planet where people still live that way. And they are thriving, too. Some argue that, while our ancestors may have thrived, their average life expectancy was half of that in the modern, industrialized world. While it is true that, on average, they may have lived shorter lives, those who died early typically died at birth, or as young adults from trauma and infection. This significantly skews the data on average life expectancy. Most of those who lived past the age of fifteen made it well into their fifties and sixties and did not die of heart disease, diabetes, and cancer the way we now do. Also those who lived to a ripe old age were still vibrant contributors—not a suffering, overmedicated, disabled tax on their community.[40]

There is no doubt that living more naturally takes hard work and dedication. I am not suggesting that we must become a hunter-gatherer society again. I am simply saying that if we can learn which characteristics of our natural environment add to our health (i.e. the food we should eat, the communities we should live in, and the type of exercise we get daily), we can begin to reclaim our health as a species. Because, just as sickness doesn't come from one missed day of exercise or one bad meal, health doesn't come from joining a gym or eating one salad. It takes personal discipline and consistent attention, and it is worth it.

So, is the lifestyle you've been living worth the price you're paying? Or, are you willing to at least consider moving in a new direction? My Be Fit, Be Nourished, Be Balanced program is a practical multistep approach to solving your lifestyle imbalances. It is based on many of the most successful recommendations we have made to our patients. While it may not be all-encompassing, the solutions outlined in this program are certainly enough to help you understand how to keep moving toward wellness on your personal health continuum for years to come.

CASE STUDY: THE BODY CAN HEAL ITSELF IN THE PROPER ENVIRONMENT.

Kristen, a thirty-nine-year-old female, was referred to our office for relief of her seasonal allergy symptoms, including itchy, watery eyes, scratchy throat, congested sinuses, and headaches. She also admitted to feeling overwhelmed at work because of constant deadlines. After reviewing her diet we found that it was high in refined carbohydrates, sugar, and refined corn products like corn syrup, high-fructose corn syrup, maltose, and dextrin. Sugar and sugar-like chemicals, like those in abundance in Kristen's diet, weaken the immune system dramatically. Kristen also ate processed foods with many preservatives, flavor enhancers, and food coloring. She had a glass of milk every morning, which would be followed by an increase in her stuffiness and mucus production.

We put her through our dietary changes and lifestyle modifications, beginning in January, typically her most allergy-free month. By the fall of the same year, she reported feeling 30 percent better than she had in the previous few years. By the end of the following summer she was symptom free and then had the best fall season she could remember.

Obviously allergies are very common, and there are many different allergens in the environment. Seasons affect each of us in our own way, and there are a host of reasons that some people are affected by allergens more than others. But in my practice we don't just treat the allergies themselves. We make sure our patients have all the nutrients their bodies require to be healthy while also removing as many potential stressors from within, as well. Then their bodies can take care of the rest.

CHAPTER SEVEN

HOW HEALTHY ARE YOU?

—

Maybe you are one of the millions of people who don't feel as well as they would like to. Maybe you feel fine, but are you healthy? Are you sick? How can you know for sure? The chart below represents your health as a continuum, ranging from very unhealthy on the left, to ideal health on the right.

0 --- 1 0 --- 2 0 --- 3 0 --- 4 0 --- 5 0 --- 6 0 --- 7 0 --- 8 0 --- 9 0 --- 1 0 0
VERY UNHEALTHY | VERY POOR | POOR | BORDERLINE | TRANSITION | GOOD | IDEAL HEALTH

It's important to realize that your location on the continuum is constantly changing in small or large increments. Each decision you make every day pushes you either a little to the left or a little to the right. The key to good health is to make as many decisions as possible that move you toward ideal health and as few as possible moving you toward sickness and death. While it would be unrealistic to always make only healthy decisions, even if 51 percent of your choices were positive, you would still gradually move yourself in a healthy direction.

If you are one of the millions of people who don't feel that well, chances are you have some kind of health issue or you are gradually moving toward the left on the continuum. You may not have received a diagnosis yet, but with consistent movement to the left, a diagnosis is inevitable.

But what if you feel fine? And what about people who feel fine but are actively engaged in poor health behaviors? Most people think that if they feel good, they are healthy. If we feel well, it's likely that we don't have any noticeable symptoms. And, of course, many people who feel well are, in fact, perfectly fine. But believing you are *healthy* because you don't have symptoms of illness may be a misconception. It can also be an incredibly dangerous premise by which to live.

Here's an example of what I mean: We all know someone who has had a heart attack. Currently, heart disease is the number one killer in the United States.[41] The symptoms of a heart attack are left arm pain, jaw pain, difficulty breathing, chest pain, profuse sweating, and fatigue. But what is really happening when you're displaying those symptoms? Right, you're having a heart attack! In other words, the first sign of a heart attack *is* a heart attack. Furthermore, for most people, there is no clear, definitive warning of an impending heart attack, as the symptoms are indications of the disease itself. That warning comes too late.

Of course, some people who have had a heart attack have also had risk factors, like high cholesterol, family history of heart disease, and high blood pressure. But many heart attack sufferers had normal cholesterol and normal blood pressure and, it turns out, these factors are not really as predictive as we once thought. If a dozen people had a heart attack today and you asked each of them how they felt the day before, very few if any of them would say they felt sick. And that isn't only true for heart attacks. It's true for virtually all chronic diseases plaguing our society, including cancers, stroke, and diabetes. It's important to understand that the way you feel—and your outward symptoms—are not always an accurate indicator of your current level of health.

So what, then, is the best indicator of health? How can you

know how healthy you are? The answer is not in how well you feel; it is in how well you function. In the following chart, select the statement from each row that best describes you.

High Function	Low Function
Usually sleep well	Usually get poor rest/sleepless nights
Typically have high energy	Often have lethargy/fatigue
Predominantly feel contentment, love, forgiveness, gratitude	Predominantly feel resentment, jealousy, anger, frustration
Able to walk or run a mile or more	Unable to walk or run a mile or more
Typically digest food properly	Often have indigestion, gastroesophageal reflux (GERD), irritable bowel syndrome (IBS)
At least one bowel movement daily	Often have constipation or diarrhea, bloating/gas
Feel in control emotionally	Often overwhelmed and overemotional
Feel energized after meals	Feel sleepy and foggy after eating
Are comfortable in your own skin	Not comfortable with your body
Notice strong new growth of hair and nails	Hair and nails do not grow quickly and/or break or crack often
Routine dental and medical exams are uneventful	At each medical or dental visit, you are told you aren't as healthy as you could be
Normal hip to waist ratio	Abnormal hip to waist ratio
Typically pain free	Chronic achiness or pain

It may be obvious to you that anyone who checks off the boxes in the left-hand column is doing very well and is probably healthy. But you may be surprised that some of the descriptions in the right-hand column could mean you're not doing very well in terms of your long-term health. Many people think symptoms in the right-hand column are indicative of normal aging. But while they are common, they are *not* normal. They may appear routine, especially since people tend to exhibit more and more of these symptoms as they age, but it is not "normal" to feel this way, regardless of your age.

If your symptoms are mostly in the right-hand column, you may be wondering, "Am I sick?" The answer is *maybe*, or *maybe not, yet.* Certainly, your body is showing signs of dysfunction, and chances are if you aren't sick today, you may be in the not-too-distant future. These symptoms are warning signs that your body is attempting to adapt to its environment. Dysfunction or "dis-ease" will always precede full-blown disease in these chronic situations. The key is for you to recognize these subtle signs, understand that they are a result of decades worth of dysfunctional lifestyle choices, and intervene with lifestyle changes immediately before the conditions get to a point where they are too advanced to be corrected.

Many who take this test do not believe they can achieve the descriptions on the left. They are so deeply entrenched in their current lifestyle that they really, truly believe that today's world simply doesn't allow for anything other than what they are now doing and experiencing. Many people comment, too, that they do not have the time or the energy to make such changes in their lives. Even when they are told their choices are setting them up for long-term illness, they don't think they can change their behavior. They believe modern life makes the list on the left impossible. But, is it *really* impossible?

It's true that to improve your health, you must learn new approaches, new thought patterns, new belief systems, and new behaviors. You must find the time, energy, and desire to work at using those new approaches, new thought patterns, and new behaviors day after day until they become your new daily habits. So no, it is *not* impossible. Of course, there will be ups and downs, but sticking with it will move your location on the continuum toward health and wellness. The most difficult part is starting the process. But once you are moving in the right direction, momentum will keep you going.

The key is to make small changes you are comfortable with. Many people who jump in headfirst find out the changes were too drastic and bounce right back in the other direction. You've probably seen this with diets and weight loss. People make a few dramatic changes and lose five, ten, or even forty pounds. But, within a span of months, all the hard work is lost and the weight comes right back because the changes were too difficult to sustain. This creates emotional stress, in addition to failing to solve the weight issue.

My advice is simple: If you keep doing what you're doing, you will keep getting what you've got. By now you've probably heard the famous saying, "The definition of insanity is doing the same thing over and over and expecting different results." So, if you *want* different results, if you want to feel different tomorrow than you do today, it's important to recognize that you're going to have to *do* different things. If this sounds daunting or overwhelming, just remember that if you keep doing what you're doing and lose your health, life is going to be a lot more daunting and a lot more overwhelming because you're not going to have your strength, your vigor, or your good health to fall back on.

When I think about my patients, whether they are my sicker patients or healthier patients, it's clear that chronic disease takes just as much hard work and commitment as good health does. And no, I'm not joking. You can either work hard every day making choices that make you sick (and probably make your family sick as well), or you can work hard every day creating health and wellness for you and your family. Remember, *your body wants to be healthy*. If you're willing to make healthy choices, let go of unhealthy habits, and create a healthy lifestyle, the dividends can be enormous. The *choice* is yours.

CASE STUDY: ADDRESSING THE BIG PICTURE, NOT JUST THE SYMPTOMS.

Debra, a fifty-four-year-old female, originally came into our office for neck tension and headaches she associated with "too much stress." After a few weeks of treatments, I asked her to bring in her latest blood work from the annual physical she'd had three months prior. This blood work showed elevated cholesterol, elevated triglycerides, and an elevated sugar panel. I explained that her stress was not only responsible for her tension and her headaches but that inside her body it was also creating an inflammatory environment of heart disease and diabetes. "Stress" does not only come from the way you feel (emotionally) but also comes from what you do to your body physically (e.g. posture, work, and sleep positions) and what you do to your body chemically (e.g. food, medications, chemicals).

We put her through a plan of dietary changes, supplements, exercise, and stress management. Within three months her cholesterol markers began to balance to a normal range. Six months later the sugar and cholesterol markers were all within normal limits. Most important, Debra felt like herself again. She felt in control of her tension and ahead of her stress.

PART TWO

THE BE FIT, BE NOURISHED, BE BALANCED PROGRAM

The Be Fit, Be Nourished, Be Balanced Program has three distinct components, each addressing one of the three stressors: physical (Be Fit), chemical (Be Nourished), and emotional (Be Balanced). The components, although distinct, interact and affect one another. If you do well in one area, that success will help you to do well in the other two areas. On the other hand, if you are doing poorly in one area, it will inhibit your ability to succeed fully in any of the other components. As you learn about the Be Fit, Be Nourished, Be Balanced program, consider how each area relates to the others, and how any one area can affect the overall results you will get from the program as a whole.

For example, nearly everyone has been on a diet at one time or another. Most diets work for a little while but don't typically work for long. You lose some weight and hit a plateau, or you gain it all back and perhaps even more. Then you become dissatisfied and frustrated with the diet and likely throw in the towel. You feel like you've worked so hard to "be good" and have tried so hard to ignore the hunger pangs and not to give in to temptation—but somehow you always seem to end up right back where you started. Each time this happens, you move deeper into a "failure" mentality. Each time, you become a little more convinced that you can never win. "Diets just don't work for me" becomes your new paradigm.

Is this lack of success an issue of nutritional health because we need to eat the right foods—that's what a "diet" is all about, isn't it? That's true, of course, but couldn't it also be an issue of physical health? We're always being told, "If you want to lose weight and get healthier, you must work on both diet and exercise." Exercise is just as important as diet. We know that if we don't get our bodies moving, we'll never win the battle. So, ultimately, it becomes an issue of physical health.

But isn't it also about making choices? And about learning? Learning how to keep yourself on track, learning to be a little more patient, learning to be a little more in control of your lifestyle? Forgiving yourself for "falling off the wagon" and then getting yourself back on track? Learning that your eating behaviors are a direct result of your thoughts and beliefs is of the utmost importance if you want to be successful on your journey to wellness. If you try to change your behaviors without changing the reason for those behaviors (your beliefs), how can you ever change for the long term? Doesn't that really sound like emotional health?

All three elements of your health must work together in order for you to succeed. You can't reach your full health potential if you don't have solid nutritional health; you can't maximize your nutrition or fitness if you don't have strong emotional health; and you can't have emotional health if you don't eat or move properly. Therefore the Be Fit, Be Nourished, Be Balanced program is designed to help you reach your goals in all three areas.

CHAPTER EIGHT

BE FIT

—

Are you more active today than you were five years ago? Do you think you will be more or less active five years from now? What about today's youth? Are they more or less active than you were when you were their age? Does activity level even matter when it comes to your health and well-being?

We often hear that exercise reduces the risk of developing conditions like depression, Alzheimer's, cancer, heart disease, diabetes, and many others. Actually, a more appropriate way to view this fact is: Lack of exercise is a major cause of the development of these conditions. Studies regarding quality of movement, activity levels, neurologic development, posture and balance, bone formation and strength, heart disease, diabetes, Alzheimer's, depression, digestion, sex drive, and cancer all show that exercise provides us with the nutrients required for our brains to process information about our environment and help our bodies prevent these conditions from developing.[42] Without exercise, many of our systems cannot function properly. You need exercise to:

- Lubricate your joints
- Reduce inflammation
- Help your body process sugar effectively

- Block pain signals
- Improve bone strength
- Increase heart efficiency
- Improve immune system function
- Maintain and improve blood sugar balance
- Keep your cholesterol levels balanced
- Reduce stress
- Prevent injuries
- Increase your longevity, and
- Improve your quality of life

Like a computer, your brain is capable of tremendous amounts of work and detailed computations. And, as they say in computer science, "garbage in, garbage out." A computer, although capable of processing immeasurable data, can do nothing without first entering good information.

Human brains are very similar to computers. Your body is monitoring temperature, digestion, heart rate, blood pressure, hormone levels, and much more without any conscious awareness on your part. The more input your brain receives about the environment you are in, the better responses it can have to the dynamic demands you put on your body. Movement (exercise) is an integral part of the data your brain needs to function and do its job properly. Industrialized populations are almost entirely sedentary, meaning they spend most of their days seated or somewhat inactive. On average, most people sit for eight to ten hours a day at school or work and sleep seven to nine hours per night, leaving only five to nine hours for other activities, which typically include time spent eating and watching television, two of Americans' favorite pastimes.[43]

With rising percentages of Americans suffering from obesity, diabetes, dementia, heart disease, cancer, high blood pressure, high cholesterol, and arthritic conditions, it is sad to share with you that over 70 percent of Americans report not getting thirty minutes of light exercise, four to five days a week.[44] In conversations with hundreds of patients, I have learned that most people think exercise and an active lifestyle are luxuries, and that if they could find the time they would do more of it. But generally, they are so busy that it is difficult for them to find the time. I say exercise is not a luxury. Exercise and movement are a *necessity* of life, and without them *sickness is imminent.*

JOINT AND SPINAL HEALTH

The human body has twenty-four bones in the spine and two synovial joints per bone. With forty-eight joints, each responsible for its share of movement, it is common to have small movement pattern restrictions in our spines. Each of these restrictions limits the necessary communication with your body, as well as creates an environment of vulnerability to injury. The spine and the muscles around the spine provide a complex network of support and movement patterns necessary for protection of the nervous system, communication with the body and brain, and movement of the body. A significant portion of signals that the brain relies on for stimulation comes from your joints. Having full range of motion of your joints, especially joints in the spine, is paramount for full signals and communication of the body with the brain allowing for optimal health expression.

Making sure that your system of bones, muscles, and nerves is functioning properly helps to ensure better health and efficient nervous system communication. Periodic evaluation by a chiropractor is a necessary component of overall physical wellness. Just as you brush your teeth twice a day *and* have a dental cleaning and exam every six months, it is important to have a professional evaluate and correct any issues with your joints, muscles, and spinal movement. You might go for adjustments once a week, twice a month, every three months, or only twice a year, depending on your stress levels, diet, exercise, and the stress-reducing outlets you have created for yourself.

CASE STUDY: MY DOCTOR SAID I'M TOO OLD TO CONTINUE RUNNING.

Shari, a forty-six-year-old woman, came into our office as a referral from her personal trainer for knee and hip pain. She had been an avid runner, but because of her pain and injuries, she was told to stop running and try something else. She began to take spin classes because, at the time, she seemed to tolerate that exercise just fine.

She was coming in for treatment because now even the spinning was causing her problems and she was concerned that she would have to give that up too. "More active five years from now," she asked as she filled out our questionnaire. "How is that possible?" She would love to be more active but couldn't imagine how that might be possible for her. She had been told numerous times by doctors that her body simply could not handle this level of exercise and that she was just too old to continue.

Upon examining Shari, it was obvious to me that her knee and hip issues had begun years earlier and her body had been compensating for so long that she now had other muscle imbalances resulting from pushing through the injuries. For some reason, she was never told to have someone address her injuries in order to help them heal properly. As a result the injuries kept compounding.

Within three weeks of working with her to break down the scar tissue, increase her range of motion, and help her regain muscle balance, she was back to spin class without any problem.

After six months of treatment she was running again, totally pain free. Shari now comes in once a month for maintenance and completely understands the importance of getting her "tune up" of spinal adjustments and muscle work to maintain her desired activity level.

THE PURPOSE OF EXERCISE

How fit should you be? What fitness level is *enough*? These are good questions, and similar questions hold true to emotional and nutritional health, too. What seems possible or desirable today will be very different from what will be possible or desirable to you six months from now. Setting realistic goals and integrating small changes into your journey seems to work well.

I've reviewed numerous fitness programs and, while the specific recommendations vary, they have certain themes in common. In general, a "fit" person should be able to swim five hundred meters, run a mile in under ten minutes, and do forty to fifty push-ups, five to ten pull-ups, and forty to fifty sit-ups. These numbers and distances are simply a goal to work toward. The sample program outlined in this book will help you meet and eventually exceed these guidelines. So, if you are starting from a baseline of no exercise, our program will help you reach these fitness guidelines. If you follow the guidelines with consistency and regularity, you should surpass your goals over time and then set new ones.

The Be Fit program is about getting your body moving, and moving it properly. If you move your body effectively, you will attain your health goals. You will reach the benchmarks outlined above and perhaps even surpass them. Don't become too focused on indicators like weight changes and calories burned. Focus on the big picture: your long-term health! Try not to focus on *symptoms*. Consider this question: Are *healthy* people overweight, underweight, or the proper weight for *them*? Of course the answer is the proper weight for them. When you keep your eyes on the big picture of your health, other indicators, like weight, will fall into place.

The Be Fit program has three purposes:

1. To help you begin your fitness journey and achieve improved fitness as compared to your current fitness level.

2. To help balance the ten physical fitness skills so that your body develops more structural integrity and becomes less likely to break down or be injured.

3. To increase your flexibility and range of motion in order to feed your brain the vital physical information it requires for optimal function and health.

Appendix A presents a fitness assessment that will help you determine how to begin strength training and how to slowly progress as your strength develops. The strength training part of the program is broken down into multiple levels or progressions, which will allow you to increase your strength safely and effectively.

Once you have exhausted the benefits of my Be Fit program, I encourage you to look for other outlets for your exercise routines. You could join a gym, hire a personal trainer, or find a boot camp to participate in. Or, if you want to really challenge yourself physically, check out a CrossFit gym near you. At some point you will need further instruction in order to set new goals and continue improving your fitness.

THE TEN SKILLS OF PHYSICAL FITNESS

What is fitness? How do we define and measure our physical fitness? There are ten skills associated with true physical fitness: endurance, stamina, strength, power, flexibility, agility, coordination, balance, accuracy, and speed. If you are lacking in any one area, you are not physically fit.

Although you will not develop these ten aspects at once, I have structured a plan that will build on each skill over time until you get to a place of proficiency with each skill. As you go through the progression of exercises, you will likely find that you are stronger in some areas than others. This is to be expected. Your goal should be to improve and strengthen each skill over time

Endurance (cardiovascular exercise)

Your level of endurance is determined by your body's ability to deliver blood and oxygen to your lungs, heart, and working muscles. The more efficient this system becomes, the easier it is for your heart to do its job. Your heart should work with the least amount of effort. The more cardiovascular exercise you do, the healthier and more efficient your heart becomes. Cardiovascular exercise—simply moving your body at a reasonable pace above the resting heart rate for twenty to sixty minutes—should be done at least four days a week. You might think of your gym's treadmill, elliptical, or stair machine as typical cardiovascular choices, but cardio exercises can include rowing, biking, running, walking, and hiking, and even interval-type training.

Stamina

Stamina is the body's level of efficiency in storing, utilizing, processing, and delivering energy. Exercises used for endurance can also be used to build stamina if done through interval training, which includes short, fast bursts of effort followed by an interval of moderate intensity. Spin classes are great examples of interval training, but any combination of short, fast movements combined with moderate duration and intensity movements qualifies.

Strength

Strength is the ability to apply force. In fitness, this includes almost all weight training exercises and resistance-oriented movements. Increasing strength in your muscles also builds strength in your joints and bones, which becomes very important as a person ages and bone density becomes a concern. Push-ups, pull-ups, sit-ups, plank pose, bench press, pull-downs, curls, squats, and many more exercises fall into this category.

Power

Power is generating maximum force in minimal time. Fast or high jumping and moving heavy weights quickly are good examples of power-building exercises.

Flexibility

Flexibility is the ability of your muscles and joints to move through a full range of motion. Flexibility training should be incorporated into your exercise routine by taking yoga, Pilates, or a stretching class, and it's important to work on your flexibility daily. On days when you're not stretching in a class, I recommend incorporating a short stretching routine every morning and a second, different one every evening. These should be performed for between 8-20 minutes per day, at most.

Agility

Agility is the ability to quickly change movement pattern or direction. Imagine how a basketball player or tennis player stops and rapidly changes direction multiple times during a game or match. Playing most team sports or working on your jump-rope skills are ways to improve your agility.

Coordination

Developing coordination includes combining multiple motion patterns into one movement. Jumping rope, doing a side shuffle, skipping, doing yoga, and dancing are all examples of coordination exercises you can incorporate into your fitness routine.

Balance

Balance is your ability to control your body's position and center of gravity. Exercising on a balance beam, board, or an exercise or

BOSU ball, as well as standing on one leg or practicing yoga balancing poses, are all great ways to develop advanced balance. Plank, side plank, and handstands will also develop your sense of balance.

Accuracy

Accuracy is the ability to control a movement in a certain direction or at a certain intensity. Working with a jump rope or treadmill, or rapidly lifting your knees to your elbows are examples of accuracy.

Speed

Speed is the velocity with which you move. Cycling between certain movements or repeating a pattern of circuit training, plyometrics, sprinting, or working at intervals are great methods of developing speed.

HOW MUCH EXERCISE SHOULD YOU GET?

The type and amount of exercise you should do depends a great deal on what your health and fitness levels are today.

In a perfect world we would move almost all day long: walking, some running, lifting and moving heavy objects, climbing, pushing, and pulling randomly throughout the day. Imagine a group of hunter-gatherers. The fitness level of an *average* hunter-gatherer was equivalent to that of today's Olympic athletes in terms of both endurance and strength.[45] How do you think you would fare living among one of these tribes today? In this day and age it is much more likely you will go the gym or work out at home, so I'll focus on what types of exercises should be done to maximize the time you spend improving or maintaining your physical fitness.

First, introduce exercise into your daily routine in a way that makes you feel comfortable. A long-term goal would be a minimum of sixty to ninety minutes of "movement" five to seven days per week. This does not have to be sixty to ninety minutes of consecutive movement; it can be broken up throughout your day. It also does not have to be the exact same exercises every time you move. Your sessions can be done in a gym, at home, or outside.

Your "daily movement" may include things like walking, hiking, running, biking, or using an elliptical machine for cardiovascular endurance, and weight training or working with resistance bands for strength training. Ideally, you should get:

- Thirty to sixty minutes of endurance movement
- Twenty to forty minutes of strength movements
- Five to twenty minutes of flexibility training, and
- Five to fifteen minutes of explosive exercises.

This routine can be done five to seven days per week, selecting a variety of daily revolving exercises. By changing the movements from day to day, you will significantly impact and improve your long-term results. You will also want to change up the whole program periodically so that your body continues to be surprised and engaged with the activities you are choosing. I have included a sample plan for you, in Appendix A, which includes some basic exercises and programming details.

CHAPTER NINE

BE NOURISHED

—

Food. It's something most of us think about a lot. We ingest it at least three times a day, and many of us snack and nibble more often than that. So it follows that healthy food is something we should know very well. Yet plenty of people, even "nutritional experts," are very confused by it.

One reason for the confusion may be that there are so many choices—too many choices. There are dozens of pasta and bread varieties, plus countless kinds of crackers, cookies, and chips. Have you walked down the cereal aisle lately? Supermarkets today hardly resemble what they looked like forty years ago—even ten years ago—and our options continue to increase, especially in the interior aisles of the supermarket, where the man-made and boxed products are featured. Yet we rarely see growth on the perimeter of the market, where the produce and meat are typically presented.

The abundance of choice is complicated by aggressive, often misleading marketing by food companies trying to entice our taste buds. And, as if that isn't enough to contend with, we must sort out the conflicting information we receive from food and health "experts" in the stores and in the news. Most of us go to the store with good intentions of buying healthy products, but we often walk out with food high in calories and/or low in nutritional value. Parents, too, are frustrated because they find their children will "only eat certain foods" and, although they know that those foods are unhealthy, they feel like they have no choice but to give them whatever they will agree to eat. We need to relearn and reprogram our understanding of food, why we eat, and what food choices are healthy and appropriate for ourselves and our families!

FOOD CHOICES

If you could start over and reestablish good nutritional habits for you and your children, what would you eat? How would you identify the healthy and unhealthy foods? How would you know which are the ideal foods for you to consume if you want to be as healthy as you can be?

Humans have existed for millennia, and we have successfully inhabited almost every geographic region. Because we have endured almost every climate, we have great data to support what our species is designed to eat. Just like a wild animal in its natural habitat knows exactly what it is supposed to eat for health and survival, humans have a natural diet that our DNA is programmed to utilize and maximize for proper function and optimal health. According to Dr. Karen Becker, "One point that no one argues is that for optimal health to occur, animals must consume the foods they were designed to eat. I call this a species-appropriate diet."[46]

Before industrialized food production, all humans consumed roughly the same diet. Except in areas of extreme climate, we ate vegetables, fruit, nuts, seeds, and meat. Before we had refrigeration or freezing, we had no choice but to eat fresh or naturally preserved versions of these same foods. Since they were grown without any chemicals, you might call most of those early foods "organic" or "free range." Our ancestors occasionally consumed dairy and grains, but those foods were not the dietary staple they are today. So, while sources of nutrition may have differed depending on our ancestors' geographical locations, the food groups that humans ate for thousands of years were essentially the same.

It's been only since the agricultural revolution that our food choices have begun to change, but even more specifically in the last one hundred to two hundred years since the industrial revolution that we've seen such a dramatic change in the foods we eat. Natural, fresh, organic, and free-range foods have only recently been replaced by manufactured, processed, genetically modified, chemically preserved, and frozen foods. In fact, the supermarket did not even exist until the early twentieth century.

Do you know what else did not commonly appear in humans until the twentieth century? Chronic lifestyle disease. According to a study published in the *New England Journal of Medicine*, "Physicians and nutritionists are increasingly convinced that the dietary habits adopted by western society over the past one hundred years make an important etiologic contribution to coronary heart disease, hypertension (high blood pressure), diabetes, and some types of cancer."[47] Not only are illnesses like heart disease, cancer, stroke, diabetes, cholesterol issues, blood pressure issues, depression, ADD/ADHD, GERD, and IBS increasingly common, they have been developing earlier and earlier in people's lives. We now have children developing early stage heart disease and type 2 diabetes, which have typically been diseases of middle age and older adults.[48]

Lifestyle disease has spread through industrialized nations like an epidemic. Since humans thrived on fresh fruit, vegetables, nuts, seeds, and lean meats for thousands of years, why wouldn't it be a good idea to eat that way now? We can continue eating processed, frozen, genetically modified, chemically altered food, and thus continue to lower the quality of our lives with epidemic rates of diabetes, cancer, and heart disease. Or, we can choose to make some sensible changes in our diets and return to feeding our bodies the fuel they want and desperately need.

The biggest issue with these changes is convenience. Healthier foods are not as readily available at your local fast-food establishment as unhealthy foods are. So, planning ahead is key. If you plan your meals effectively, carry healthy snacks with you on a regular basis, and feed yourself consistently throughout the day, you will be successful making the changes required to get and stay healthy.

Patients often ask me, "If food today is so bad for us and the food of our past was so good for us, why are we living longer today than ever?" This is a great question, and one with a few answers. First, although life expectancy has increased to age seventy-seven, quality of life remains at approximately age sixty. We live longer in spite of the chronic lifestyle diseases because we use surgery and medication to control the damage. Among our hunting and gathering ancestors it was not uncommon to have people live well into their sixties. As mentioned earlier, "average" life expectancy was low in those communities because many members died in childbirth or very young from infection or trauma.[49] More important, those who did live into their sixties maintained a consistently high quality of life until death. They did not spend their last one or two decades living with the disease, organ failure, or the loss of function we see today. Although our life expectancy and high quality of life is similar today as it was then, if we took better care of ourselves, our life expectancy would continue to increase and, I believe, our quality of life index would skyrocket as well.

FOOD QUANTITY

There is, of course, another growing problem, particularly here in the US and other industrialized countries. You may have heard or noticed that we not only have a *quality* of food issue, but we also have a *quantity* of food issue. Most of us know that if we eat more we will weigh more. But what is also true and frequently overlooked is that when we weigh more, we need to eat more. Many people are not aware of this, nor that this concept is used and abused by many, if not all, food manufacturers and distributors.

Food companies know that if they can get you to eat just a little more, you will gain a little more weight. In turn you will need more food to maintain your metabolism and curb your hunger. Then, the next time you visit the grocery store or fast food chain, you will buy even more food. And the cycle continues. From this pattern, the idea of the "supersize" meal was born to satisfy the hunger for larger quantities of food—certainly not to help you save money or stay fit.

I ask my patients, "How many potato chips can you eat?" (The question could apply to pretzels, popcorn, ice cream, doughnuts, or any other low-nutrient, high-calorie food product.) Invariably the answer is "a lot." That stuff goes down very easily and, before you know it, you've eaten a whole bag of chips, a half-gallon of ice cream, or half a dozen donuts. That's a lot of food—a lot of nutritionally poor food, to boot.

Why are you able to eat so much bad-for-you food? Many food manufacturers alter the taste of foods so that you keep eating. There are whole teams in food development devoted to keeping your taste buds excited enough to crave and consume as much of these foods as possible. Another reason we can consume so much unhealthy food is that we have two physical mechanisms for hunger and satiety. First is the capacity of the stomach organ to expand and contract as food fills it; the second is the absorption of nutrients from the meal. If you eat a whole bag of potato chips you will start to feel one type of fullness, such as bloating, distending, or nausea from the stretching of your stomach. But you won't feel satisfied! You may even still be slightly hungry. You are not satisfied because there were tons of calories and other "stuff" in that large quantity of "food" you ingested, but there were no nutrients. You did not satisfy your nutrient need, so your body is looking for more.

On the other hand, let's say I give you a nice shiny, crunchy apple. You eat the whole apple down to the core. Would you want another one? Probably not. But let's say you do eat a second apple, would you ever consider a third? No way. That's because you've taken in more than enough nutrients from the apple. Even more important, would you be distended, bloated, or nauseated? No. You can feel fully satisfied well before your stomach is actually full by eating low-calorie, highly nutritious foods. It's very unlikely that you will ever feel satisfied by eating high-calorie, low-nutrient junk food no matter how much you eat. A lack of satisfaction from the food we eat and from our lives has caused a severe overeating epidemic in this country. As a result, obesity rates are increasing alongside other lifestyle diseases.

We must get back to basics with our food. Although this is easy to explain and should be easy to understand, it may seem difficult to make the changes in your diet. We know that fresh food is healthier than processed food. And now you know why you feel the way you do about the foods you often crave and eat. So why aren't you able to do what you know you should in order to keep yourself healthy? It boils down to your emotional health, which will be addressed in chapter 10, "Be Balanced." You know you should not eat that brownie because it will contribute to weight gain and you'll have to run six extra minutes tomorrow to make up for consuming the extra calories. Those are the immediate consequences, but they're just the tip of the iceberg. The damage going on inside your body from the unhealthy food choices you are making is devastating. When you fully understand these consequences you will make different decisions.

Here is another analogy from Dr. Chestnut to illustrate the point: Pizza is one of the most commonly overeaten foods in the United States. It is high in calories, low in nutrient content, and contains two of the three categories of ingredients (wheat and dairy) on what I call my "limit/eliminate food list." If you're like most people, I'm sure you would gladly eat a slice or two. What if I told you the slice is poisoned? Would you still eat it? It would look the same, taste the same, and feel the same. The only difference would be the poison. You wouldn't eat it, would you? Of course not!

Well, if you understood how the food you ate affected your health, you would understand that the pizza was slowly poisoning you. You would understand that the ingredients of that pizza are inflammatory, that a high-wheat diet will push your health toward obesity, diabetes, and heart disease, and that the dairy likely contained antibiotics, hormones, and other unknown chemicals. If you looked at pizza from this viewpoint, you would think twice and choose something else, right? That doesn't mean you can never have another slice of pizza, but it should make you reconsider it as a lunch or dinner option on a regular basis.

All food can be categorized as one of three macronutrients: carbohydrates, fats, or proteins. If you currently eat a lot of one macronutrient and you decide to remove that entire macronutrient from your diet (e.g., the Atkins Diet removing carbohydrates), you will lose weight. But you will not become healthier. You need to incorporate specific substrates found in certain foods in order to improve your health. While removing certain types of food from your diet may help you lose weight, it may also shift you in the direction of sickness rather than health. Also, you will be dissatisfied with these new restrictions in your diet. Dissatisfaction with your new diet will always lead you to giving up. As I mentioned previously, each time you give up it moves you deeper into a "failure" mentality. Learning why you should make certain choices is just as important—if not more important—than actually making the right choices.

To help you make healthy choices, I have compiled a list of foods to increase in your diet, as well as ingredients to identify and avoid in food labels. I encourage you to examine food labels and get an idea of what you are eating. See where you might begin to limit your intake of unhealthy ingredients.

WATER

While there are many different foods that your body requires for optimal health, there is only one necessary liquid: water. The human body is 60 to 70 percent water.[50] You cannot survive more than one to two weeks without water, and most people are partially dehydrated all the time.

Some people claim to love water while others say they do not care for it much. Whether you like water or not, you must drink it; your body requires it to function properly. While many of the drinks we consume are "mostly" water with some type of additive, it is important to drink water all by itself, too. Fresh lemon, lime, or cucumber added to your water is perfectly fine, but adding sugar or artificial sweeteners and drinking soda, tea, or coffee does not count as a "water" choice.

In this context it is important to define diuretics. Diuretics pull water out rather than add water to your body. Coffee and some teas are among the most commonly consumed diuretics. I usually suggest you drink eight ounces of water for every eight ounces of coffee or tea (one cup) to ensure you do not get dehydrated.

A good general rule is that your body requires forty-eight to sixty ounces (six to eight cups) of water every day, and more if you are consuming any diuretic beverages.

FOODS

Your diet should include 65 to 75 percent plant-based foods (fruits, vegetables, nuts, and seeds) and 25 to 35 percent healthy animal protein (grass-fed beef, wild-caught fish, free-range and organic pork, poultry, and eggs).

Many patients ask about vegan and vegetarian diets. Although humans are omnivores, meaning they can survive on almost any food product, there are certain foods that allow your health to flourish. In my research, it is clear that animal protein is a necessary component of the human diet. Healthy lean meat is an important source of naturally occurring B vitamins, fats, oils, iron, and amino acids—all of which your body requires for the proper functioning of the brain, nervous, cardiovascular, and immune systems, as well as energy production systems.

Many studies conflict on the topic of meat in the diet, but I believe most of this information is skewed and misinterpreted. There's a theory that if humans eat meat from sick animals (and most meat today comes from unhealthy and over-medicated animals), we should expect that meat to make us sick, and that makes sense to me. There are plenty of other studies to show that humans in hunting populations who eat healthy, wild animals have little or no increase in inflammation, heart disease, or stroke. That theory also makes sense to me. I agree that most Americans consume too much animal protein and not nearly enough vegetables. But, if we consume *healthy* animal products in respectable quantities, we should expect *healthy* results. Being a vegan or vegetarian for moral or ethical reasons is completely understandable; however, I do not believe that vegan or vegetarian diets are superior from a health perspective.

FOODS TO EAT AND FOODS TO ELIMINATE

Human DNA, or genetic code, is programmed to require certain foods in order to produce all of our hormones and neurotransmitters, as well as to generate new cells to repair and maintain a strong body and mind. If you are eating too little of these healthy foods, or eating too much unhealthy food, your body will not function properly, let alone optimally.

What Should We Be Eating?

- Filtered water
- Organic fruits and vegetables (mostly raw, but some cooked is okay, too)
- Grass-fed, antibiotic-free, organic, free-range meat, chicken, and fish
- Organic and raw nuts, seeds, and *some* legumes (in limited quantities)
- Healthy oils like fish, flax, olive, and coconut

Foods to Eat Sparingly, If at All

The following list presents foods that have damaging effects on your health and physiology, and your consumption of these foods should be very limited or eliminated completely. These foods create inflammation, are potentially toxic, and any possible nutritional benefit could easily be realized by eating other healthier foods. When consumed in moderate-to-high quantities, these foods decrease your health, your life span, and your quality of life.

- Wheat (all wheat-flour-based products like bread, sandwiches, pizza, cookies, cakes, muffins, etc.)
  - Wheat can cause greater blood sugar spikes than actual sugar itself. It is an inflammatory food and is often responsible for stomach bloating, gas, and other gastrointestinal issues. The potential to push you toward heart disease, cholesterol imbalances, autoimmune diseases, diabetes, and cancer from wheat are high.

- Dairy from cows (including whey, casein, and lactose products)
  - All mammals drink milk, and humans are no exception. But no other mammal drinks milk past infancy and, more important, no mammal drinks another mammal's milk

except for humans. So milk does have its function with humans, but we have taken that to a whole new level.

- Milk is a common allergen and often the cause of excessive mucus production. In addition, if the dairy product is not organic, it will have originated with cows injected with high levels of antibiotics and hormones used to prevent diseases from their poor living conditions and to keep them lactating. When you consume the milk or dairy products from these cows, you are also consuming those drugs.

- Soy (including soy beans, vegetable oil, soy protein, and soy lecithin)

  - Soy is one of the most common genetically modified organism (GMO) foods we consume, and at this time there is no real data to support any health benefit. On the contrary, studies are coming out that seem to show many health consequences of genetic engineering. Based on my research, I recommend avoiding all GMOs whenever possible.

  - Soy has a strong estrogenic effect; it is a common allergen and is an inflammatory food even in its purest form. As a result, soy should be considered dangerous and not a health food as it once was touted to be.

- Corn (corn syrup, high fructose corn syrup, vegetable oil, maltose, dextrin, and xanthan gum)

  - Corn has become an issue recently because corn syrup, its processed by-product, is a common ingredient in many packaged foods and beverages, including soft drinks, milk, candy, and baked goods. The processing corn goes through to make it a syrup sweetener also makes it a common allergen and an ingredient in foods that contribute to increases in obesity, diabetes, and heart disease.

- Corn on the cob may not be a dangerous food on its own, as long as it has not been genetically modified (GMO), but consumption should still be very limited.

- Peanuts

  - Peanuts are legumes, not nuts. Peanuts are often contaminated with a mold called aflatoxin, a very common allergen and neurotoxin (brain and nerve poison). The anaphylactic peanut allergy is becoming more and more prevalent in children. Any real nut and/or nut butter, including almond, cashew, and sunflower seed, is a better choice.

- Dried fruit

  - Drying the fruit concentrates the natural sugars, making dried fruit very high in sugar per serving.

  - The drying process often utilizes preservatives, such as sulfites, to make their shelf life much longer. Homemade dried fruit or dried fruit without strong chemical preservatives may be consumed in small quantities.

- Caffeine

  - Caffeine is a stimulant. It is a drug, and much like sugar, most industrialized nations are addicted to both. Caffeine may lower our ability to tolerate sugar levels by lowering our insulin sensitivity and directly affecting our bodies' ability to manage stress.

- Fruit juices

  - Fruit juices contain highly concentrated sugar levels. Their processing and storage (added coloring and sugar; pasteurization) make them undesirable and unhealthly. Homemade, fresh juice may be consumed in small to moderate amounts.

Foods to Eliminate

The following foods should be eliminated. These foods contain chemicals that have been proven to cause or at least contribute to health problems and will certainly move you to the left on the health continuum.[51]

- Fried foods

- Processed foods

- Foods treated with pesticides

- Artificial sweeteners

  ○ Chemical sweeteners, such as saccharine, acesulfame potassium, aspartame, sucralose, and neotame, are potentially toxic and known to increase rates of cancer and/or neurologic diseases.

  ○ They also cause a "sugar" response, similar to that of real sugar, within the body. They also stimulate cravings for increased consumption of food.

- All trans fats

  ○ Trans fats are essentially rancid oils that cause inflammation, an increase in LDL (bad cholesterol), and a decrease in HDL (good cholesterol).

- Hydrolyzed proteins, also known as MSG

  ○ Hydrolyzed proteins are common food additives used to heighten food flavor, thus exciting the brain and making us crave more of those foods. Hydrolyzed proteins are considered a neurotoxin (nerve and brain toxin).

- All genetically modified foods. Look for labels that say "Non-GMO."

- Preservatives and artificial coloring and flavoring

  ○ There are a variety of preservatives, artificial colors, and artificial flavors found in the foods stocked on the super-market interior aisles. The chemicals in preservatives and artificial coloring and flavoring range from inflammatory to toxic to carcinogenic. Although deemed safe enough in small dosages by the FDA, the safety of food additives is questionable at best and certainly contribute nothing beneficial to your overall health.

- Grain-fed, hormone-, and antibiotic-treated meats. Consuming such animal products can cause human illness.

BEHAVIORS TO LIVE BY

People are not very mindful when they eat. If a snack is left out on a table or desk they'll pick at it. If they have a particular craving they will satisfy it. Most weight issues stem from people mindlessly fulfilling their own cravings. I encourage you to become more conscious about your choices. Here is an exercise to help you:

For at least two weeks straight, ask yourself these two questions before you put anything in your mouth:

1. Why am I eating this food?

2. Is this food going to make me healthier or make me sicker?

Is it because it's time to eat and you are hungry? Or is it because you are stressed, wanting comfort, bored, or just being social? The answers to these questions will help you understand why you are eating whatever you are eating.

This exercise also gives you the opportunity to assess which direction on the health continuum the food will move you in. After asking yourself these questions you might still decide to eat that food regardless of the answers. That's okay; at least you will be more conscious about the choice. In the long term, this exercise may help you say no to certain foods or certain situations.

Meal Plan

As you discover meals and food ideas that appeal to you, start collecting them in a list. It is very easy to eat consciously and healthy when you plan your meals ahead of time. If you plan your meals and your meal times, you can avoid getting yourself into a situation where unhealthy choices are your only alternative. If you carry healthy snacks with you all the time—for when you find yourself away from home and starving—this practice may help you avoid eating something unhealthy.

Shopping

Here are three important, easy-to-follow rules for food shopping:

1. Never go to the grocery store hungry. I'm sure you have made impulse buys at the grocery store. Many unhealthy food items would not make it home if people did not shop on an empty stomach.

2. Shop the perimeter (but not the bakery!). Since most packaged foods fill the middle aisles, keeping to the perimeter of the store increases your chances of shopping successfully.

3. If you don't bring it home, you can't eat it!

CHAPTER TEN

BE BALANCED

—

If your health is a product of your choices, it's important for you to realize that making a choice is primarily an *emotional* process. You take in the information, list and evaluate the pros and the cons (on both the conscious and unconscious levels), and then . . . you decide to eat an entire bag of cookies during a long night of watching TV. Oops! What happened?

The reason you make an unhealthy choice despite knowing it's bad for you is that you have trouble connecting your actions with what the consequences will be. We all know that eating unhealthy food and getting little or no exercise will not make us healthier. But, in the moment, when you're struggling to make a choice, you just want to satisfy a craving. You don't stop to think about how unhealthy that choice really is or evaluate the long-term consequences of making that choice. Since everything is interrelated, every choice you make has a consequence, but each of your decisions will also affect your other choices. A common example of this is, "Well I already ate a cookie; I might as well try the brownies and cake, too."

Take Bill, for example. One evening, Bill has an argument with his wife and they go to bed without resolving their issues. He doesn't sleep well that night. He wakes up feeling groggy and stressed. He may even sleep through his alarm and be late for work. He has no time to make breakfast and isn't thinking about taking care of himself—that's the last thing on his mind. So, instead of having a healthy breakfast, Bill stops on the way to work and grabs a donut and a cup of coffee. Between the sugar rush and the caffeine, he's not at his best for the client presentation that morning. He starts to worry if his bad performance will affect his job security. Very quickly, Bill finds himself in a downward spiral. And, if he wasn't in the best of health to begin with, he could actually be headed for some real health problems if he keeps this up.

Now, let's take a look at Sam, who has an argument with his wife one evening, but before going to bed, he remembers to spend a few minutes writing in the journal he's been keeping for a few months. It's become a habit for him to jot down a few things he's thankful for every night at bedtime. He writes things like the fact that he has a job that helps support his family, that he and his wife own their own home, and that they have two kids he's proud of. As he is writing after the fight, Sam begins to think that he might have been a little unreasonable when he was arguing with his wife earlier that evening. He decides that he should try to talk with her a little more before they go to sleep.

He asks her to restate the point she was trying to make because he's not sure he fully understood what she was trying to say. She then tries to restate her point in a way that Sam can relate to. Reminded that he's thankful to have a wife like her, he apologizes for being unreasonable. Once she feels like she has been understood, Sam has a chance to restate his opinion and they discuss the issue in a calm, active-listening manner. Stephen Covey, author and educator, sums up this process perfectly: "Seek first to understand, then to be understood."

When Sam returns to bed, his stress level is low. He's feeling pretty good. He sleeps well and wakes up a few minutes before the alarm the next morning. He has a healthy breakfast and takes a walk around the neighborhood before going to the office. He uses this walking time to mentally prepare for the presentation he needs to make that morning. When he gets to work, he's ready for his client presentation and he does a great job.

What Sam did is not difficult. People often think they must move to a desert island to be free of stress. But the truth is you can just as effectively lower your stress level today—right here, right now. It is all about preparation and timing. One easy way to achieve this is to take a deep breath and think about the good things in your life. Thinking good, positive thoughts—thoughts about gratitude, love, and forgiveness—has a positive effect on your stress immediately, and those effects accumulate over time. Why is this an important action? If you're blessed with positive feelings, if you're feeling loved, if you're feeling forgiveness toward others, you're more likely to make more positive, healthy decisions about other important things in your life—like what you eat and how much you exercise.

About forty years ago, Thomas Holmes and Richard Rahe conducted a landmark study about stress. This study showed the connection between stress levels and likelihood of illness. The average American at that time had a stress level of 150. All things being equal, that level carries a relatively low likelihood of illness. However, Holmes and Rahe found that if a person had a level of 300, that person would have a 90 percent chance of developing a serious illness within a year, leading not only to a high chance of getting very sick, but also of being hospitalized.[52] That's right, 90 percent!

How do you get to a stress level of 300? Usually, it takes a series of major stresses to reach that number. Lose a job and get divorced and you're on your way. But it can also be a series of smaller stresses much like the ones Americans face every day. Work long hours in an unpleasant job with a nasty boss, inhale some fast food for dinner, and come home to a cramped apartment and an irritable spouse, and you'll find yourself becoming very sick at some point.

But you need that job, right? So what are you supposed to do?

It's all about your attitude. There will always be situations in life that can make you miserable. Work is hardly ever going to be as much fun as vacation. Relationships will never always be smooth sailing. Although you can't control everything that goes on in your life, you can control the way you think about those things. As Francesca Reigler famously said, "Happiness is an attitude. We either make ourselves miserable, or happy and strong. The amount of work is the same."

A nasty boss, a bad marriage, or a traumatic situation can be extremely painful. No amount of attitude adjustment is going to change that, but choosing to be miserable about it only makes a bad situation worse. Too often, people ignore the tools that are available to deal with the challenging aspects of life. You have friends or counselors you can talk to. You can make time to get away, take a break, or clear your head. You can get some exercise, learn to meditate, or do one of the dozens of endorphin-producing activities that can ease the pain and help you to heal, such as learning a new hobby, going for a hike, or spending quality time with your family. Then you are better able to step back from the ledge of pain and misery and find the energy to choose a different response. Put your energy into things you have control over; try not to become overwhelmed with what you cannot control in your life. As Mary Engelbreit said, "If you don't like something, change it; if you can't change it, change the way you think about it." Change your thought patterns so you can change your behaviors, and then you'll have the power to change your outcomes.

We all doubt ourselves and our situations sometimes; we all find things to complain about in ourselves, in others, and in the world around us. Unless you're a yogi or a saint, chances are good that you have a tendency toward negative thinking—not just about your own situation, but about other people and the world at large. As a health care practitioner, I've seen that negative thoughts really do have negative health consequences. Just like the effects of eating unhealthy food, negative thinking adds up over time. Picture this: You're driving down the road, traffic isn't bad, and you're on track to get to your meeting on time. Then brake lights appear as far as the eye can see. Panic begins to set in as you slow down to a crawling five miles an hour. You don't know if there's been an accident or if it's just high volume, and the traffic report on the radio doesn't mention the road you're on. You're in the dark about what's going on, and you're stuck.

So, how do you prevent yourself from going down the path of negative thinking? First, take a deep breath. Better yet, take a few deep, slow breaths. You might be surprised how that simple act can change your attitude. Deep breathing tends to usher in a new perspective. Then take stock of the situation by asking yourself a series of questions:

- How important is it that you get to your destination on time?
- How late can you be without major consequences?
- Is there another route you can take to avoid the traffic?
- Is there someone you can call who can explain the situation?
- And finally: Is this a life or death situation? Or are you overreacting?

If you find that your thinking is borderline catastrophic, remind yourself of all the catastrophes you've feared before in your life that haven't come to pass. So there's a good reason to think that this latest one won't amount to very much either.

Try to find a good side to the situation. Use the time to take a look around you. Maybe you're on a parkway or a highway surrounded by trees, clouds, or a beautiful blue sky. Open your car window, take one more deep breath, and listen to the birds. When I'm stuck in traffic I choose to accept it as a lesson in patience. I try to use the time to think about the rest of my day and problem-solve other tasks on my plate. Whether this shift in perspective works the first time, the second time, or not until the twentieth time, don't give up. Keep trying! Staying positive and relaxed in the face of stress can take time and requires practice. Enjoy the journey. When you can master this, healthy thinking will become easier to apply to other areas of your life, like your daily diet.

I have examined many diet and exercise programs and, in my opinion, none of them were designed for success. Why? Because they only tell you what to do, not how to think about what you're doing or, more important, lay the groundwork for *why* you are doing it. You cannot modify your behavior until you modify your beliefs. Your actions are a direct result of your thoughts, and your thoughts are only your thoughts because of your belief system. If your belief system is "I hate exercise," it does not matter how many times someone tells you to do it, you won't, illustrating that your actions will be in line with the belief that you do not like it. That belief must change before you can see lasting changes in your behavior. Whether you do or do not like to exercise, a belief system in which you value your health and your ability to play with your children, for example, creates thoughts that are more likely to get you to exercise in order to become healthier.

Try not to beat yourself up if you get off track; learn to forgive yourself. We all get off track from time to time. It's essential to pick yourself up and get right back on. Forgive your own mistakes every chance you get. Then try to forgive the mistakes—even the bad behaviors—of other people. Criticizing, judging, and putting down other people will not make you feel any better. Judging other people usually results in anger and negative emotions. All that negativity makes your health worse—and it will certainly make your health measurably worse over time. When you can do this, you'll notice how quickly your stress levels will come down. Good health might not come easily at first. Keep practicing, though, and watch it get easier over time.

FINDING BALANCE

Developing proficiency with any new skill requires practice. Establishing, maintaining, and improving your emotional health is no exception. Through repetition, your brain learns thought and behavior patterns, and the way you respond to situations, handle emotional stress, build relationships, and tolerate adversity have been created over your lifetime through your experiences. Often when presented with a difficult situation, a person will react a certain way and then think later, "I wish I would have said *this* instead," or, "I could have done *that* differently." Then days, weeks, or months later a similar situation arises and they handle it the same exact way. Why is this? It happens again and again because you didn't practice the outcome you wanted. It's analogous to an athlete never showing up for practice and on game day running the wrong plays. If you do not practice the skills you want to develop, how can you expect to have different outcomes? As I discussed earlier, your belief system is the catalyst for your thoughts. Your thoughts generate your behavior patterns.

A crucial step in rebuilding your health is to control your beliefs and your thoughts. When your thoughts are not in line with your goals, behavioral change is difficult. If, however, your thoughts *are* in line with your goals, transitions are easier and behavior changes become automatic. Therefore, I recommend working on belief and thought changes first. Here are eleven principles that will help you think in a healthier, more constructive way. If you can apply these principles to your life, you'll be making a good start down the road to better health.

SET YOUR COMPASS

As Dr. James Chestnut teaches, "Your values are your compass." You can call on your compass (your values) whenever you must make a decision. Once you have determined your values (honesty, dedication, determination, being team-oriented, being open minded, etc.), "doing the right thing" becomes your default. You become very clear on what to do and how to handle tough situations. Ask yourself questions such as: What is important to me? What attributes do I want to possess and want other people to see? Then, when presented with what seems like a major dilemma, take out your compass and see how your values line up. No matter how easy or tough the issue may be, you will not make the wrong decision if it's in line with your values. Your choices then become clear.

In addition to helping with tough situations and decisions, using your compass will also help you make positive health-related decisions. If your health is high on your value list, you will use your compass to make healthy lifestyle decisions as well. Perhaps you are faced with choosing between a slice of pizza or a piece of fish with grilled vegetables for lunch. Your emotional self may say, "Give me the pizza, please!" This is the exact reason that behavior changes are so difficult. If, however, you consulted your compass, it would clearly point to the fish with grilled veggies. That choice would be clear and easy to make. Changing your thoughts and beliefs first will always lead you toward changing your behavior.

IMPROVE YOUR EVENING ROUTINE

Our bodies function on a circadian rhythm that prompts the body to feel hungry, to feel tired, and to eliminate waste. When life is hectic, the circadian rhythm can get out of sorts. Insufficient sleep is associated with chronic inflammation, insulin resistance, diabetes, and obesity.[53] Practicing healthy evening routines helps to retrain your essential sleeping rhythm to get back on track, which in turn will aid in reestablishing your other essential rhythms.

In order to get back on track with your circadian rhythm, I recommend that you be consistent in your routine every night—even on the weekends. Turn off your cellular phones, computers, and televisions at least one hour before bedtime. Change your clothes and brush your teeth before you get too tired and fall asleep on the couch. (Falling asleep on the couch too early and waking up at midnight to get ready for bed is very disruptive to your rhythm.) Read, talk to your spouse, jot your thoughts down in your gratitude journal, or meditate. These actions will allow your body time to shut down after a long day and will promote better, more restful sleep.

IMPROVE YOUR MORNING ROUTINE

You may have heard of the "hour of power," a concept promoted by personal development leader Tony Robbins. The hour of power is a dedicated block of time first thing in the morning when you create, plan, brainstorm, write, organize, exercise, and/or make your day's to-do list. It may be an hour, as the name suggests, or it may be ten or fifteen minutes if that is all you can spare. This type of morning routine allows you to proactively plan your day and prepare for obstacles before they come your way. Creating a pattern of being *proactive* leads to a more relaxing and less stressful life than being *reactive* and waiting to deal with the day's issues as they appear. Reactive living is the fast track to becoming overwhelmed by stress.

Your morning hour of power sets the tone for your day and gets you ready for whatever it might bring. To develop this new routine, you may need to set your alarm fifteen or thirty minutes earlier, or maybe you can manage your morning time better. If you're a multitasker, combine some of your exercise routines like stretching and walking with your mental preparation for your day. You can create a mental list of tasks you'll accomplish or visualize how it will feel to achieve your goals that day.

Implementing an evening routine and establishing your hour of power will require time management and making clear choices. It might mean foregoing that last television show you love or hitting the snooze button only once (or, better yet, not at all) in the morning. But the quality-of-life and stress-reduction payoff you'll receive is tremendous.

DEFINE YOUR PURPOSE

Whether in your career, your personal life, or both, you *must* define your purpose. It's your reason for *being* and it drives your behavior. Defining your purpose—the why you do what you do and who you want to be—helps define what you should be *doing* to achieve your goals. Although many people know there are things they should be doing, they can easily provide many reasons (even excuses) to choose not to do them. Being clear on your purpose—even writing down your purpose statement—will increase the chances that you will choose the behaviors that take you closer to that purpose and eliminate behaviors that are keeping you from reaching your potential.

BE PRESENT

Anxiety has been described as worry about future events, while depression has been described as concern or worry about the past. Both of these conditions add a tremendous amount of stress to life and ultimately make some of these other changes more difficult. Time spent worrying about things we cannot control is wasted time and brings with it feelings of hopelessness. Coming up with ways to deal with things you *do* have control over is productive and reduces stress. When you are living in the present moment, you can neither be anxious nor depressed.

The best way to stop yourself from becoming anxious about the "what ifs" or too depressed about what was, is to be present. Try to be fully present each and every moment of your life. Bringing your full, conscious attention to each moment will prevent your mind from drifting to the unknown. This is a skill that requires practice. Check in with yourself and see how often you are truly present. Begin bringing your attention to the present moment and watch your stress decrease immediately. We all experience the most pleasure and satisfaction in our lives when we are present.

LEARN THE "BE, DO, HAVE" MODEL

Most of us have been taught to believe that once you've achieved a certain level of success you will become a certain type of person. This leads us to believe that we must *have* certain things or *do* certain things to become who we want to be. This way of thinking can be destructive, especially when people feel like they may never become who they aspire to be because they do not have the things they think they need. The "Be, Do, Have" model is exactly opposite of that destructive thinking and will help you improve your place in life. You must first *Be* (behave as if you are) the person and then *Do* the proper steps in order to *Have* whatever it is that you want. You first decide what you want to Have (determine your goal), then you create a plan of what you need to Do (map out the steps you must take to reach that goal), and then determine the type of person you need to become. Become that person and watch yourself get closer to the things you want in your life. I have found this process to be profoundly helpful for personal and professional success.

Begin with an area in your life you would like to improve. This could be your family life, your business, your job, or anything you want. Write down a no-rules, anything-goes description of your dream. (If you've never done this, it's a really fun and enlightening exercise.) Next, list the steps you must do to achieve this goal. Finally, think about the traits, attitudes, and perspective you must have to accomplish that goal. Those are the attributes you must incorporate into your life today so that you may become the person you want to be.

A simple example of this would be putting a plan together to start your own business or to achieve a promotion. As you dream about what that business and/or new job looks like, start making a list of the type of person that would make this a successful venture. Would they be dedicated to the mission of the business? Would they stop working at five o'clock or not until they completed all their tasks for the day? Would they be willing to go above and beyond for the company? Might they also be honest, trustworthy, hardworking, and have high self-esteem? Once you establish a list of attributes, start behaving in that way. Become the person you need to be in order to have access to and get the things you want.

PRACTICE FORGIVENESS

Forgiveness is one of the first steps to emotional healing. It allows you to free yourself from holding onto the negative emotions associated with a person or situation. It's not necessary for you to say, "What you did is okay," in order to forgive someone, especially if it's *not* really okay. However, you can say, "You are forgiven." This means that what someone did is not okay but that they are forgiven for the behavior. Holding a grudge forces you to relive the negative experience and allows those emotions to control your thoughts and your behaviors. Practicing forgiveness gives you more control over your thoughts and your emotions.

KEEP A JOURNAL

Keeping a gratitude journal is easy and requires only about five minutes a day. Jot down five things that you are grateful for before you go to bed or during your morning hour of power. Some entries may repeat from time to time, but try to think of at least a few new entries every day. This is a great practice for appreciating the small things in life, and it helps to ease the stress of the day.

PURSUE A HOBBY

We all need time to do what we love to do. If you're like most people, you probably used to have hobbies that you no longer participate in because your life has become too hectic or busy. Leading a proactive life frees up time for you to fill any way you'd like. When you fill your time this way, being busy becomes rewarding, fun, and not stressful. We are all busy, usually from the moment we wake up until we fall asleep. What activities you decide to fill this time with is ultimately up to you. Most people allow their time to be filled for them by what goes on around them (reactive living). By adding the fulfilling, stress-reducing habits I've suggested, you will be surprised at how much extra time you will have. This should allow you to pick up a new hobby or rediscover an old one, thus taking another step toward reaffirming that you are important. These activities should be scheduled in your life like an important meeting. It is too easy not to go to the gym, pick up the guitar, read, or knit because someone has asked you to do something else. When your hobbies are scheduled, you are committed to them. You are saying, "This is important to me and other demands must wait."

PRACTICE AFFIRMATIONS

Affirmations are positive self-talk. An affirmation can be a word, phrase, or a complete sentence, and is always said in the present tense. Affirmations can cover any aspect of your life, especially the ones in need of improvement.

You can easily find affirmations others have created on the Internet or in books, but I recommend you make them your own. Your affirmations must feel right to you in order to work properly. Generally an affirmation should begin with expectations for the day. An example is, "It's a great day!" or "I am ready to conquer the day!" or "I am excited for what today will bring and expect to be ready for whatever comes my way." The next affirmation should help you move away from things that are holding you back. For example: "I choose to let go of my fear, my self-sabotage, and my anxiety." Then state something that will move you in the direction you want to go, such as, "I choose to be confident. I am smart. I am handsome. I can solve any problem. I am a great husband and father." Especially after you understand the "Be, Do, Have" plan, affirmations will help you define and become who you want to be.

THE EMOTIONAL BANK ACCOUNT

Author Stephen Covey, in his book *The 7 Habits of Highly Effective People*, wrote about a concept he calls the "emotional bank account." He said that you must make emotional deposits with everyone before you can make a withdrawal.[54] The essential message of the emotional bank account is to give everyone the benefit of the doubt.

Create an emotional bank account for every person in your life. Give them a full account, right from the beginning. If they do something you don't like or don't appreciate, consider that a withdrawal. If they do something you do like or do appreciate, consider that a deposit. A few withdrawals taken from time to time are no big deal; we all need to make withdrawals on occasion. As long as a couple of deposits are also made, there will be a positive balance in the account. If the balance gets too low, though, either from too few deposits or too many withdrawals, it's okay to close that person's account and move on. Keep the relationships in your life positive. At the same time remember to regularly make deposits into the emotional bank accounts of the people you love and who are important to you.

SELF-ESTEEM

It is imperative that you manage your self-esteem. Do things that make you feel good about yourself, and strive to avoid things that make you feel bad. Taking care of your health is a great way to affirm for yourself that you are valuable. When your thoughts and beliefs are in line with your actions, your self-esteem will soar. When they are in contradiction, your self-esteem erodes.

Help build your loved ones' self-esteem, especially your spouse and children. I believe good parents don't spoil their kids but instill a strong sense of self and of self-worth and responsibility. If we protect our children too much or allow them to avoid taking responsibility for their mistakes, they cannot learn how to be successful adults. By investing in the self-esteem of our loved ones, we are also reinforcing our own value and building self-esteem for ourselves.

CHAPTER ELEVEN

THE CHILDREN

My greatest motivation for writing this book is our children. Not only are we experiencing a drastic decline in our health and quality of life, but even as I write this book, humans are the sickest we have ever been. Today's children are the unhealthiest generation ever. Between lack of exercise, unhealthy food choices, low self-esteem, and poor social skills, today's youth are facing serious health challenges.

Children eight years old and younger are showing signs of and being medicated for conditions that usually take decades to show up. We have never before seen these rates of obesity, high cholesterol, high blood pressure, diabetes, depression, or ADD/ADHD in children. The only effective way to treat this problem is to properly diagnose and treat its *cause*, not just its symptoms. Today's childhood health epidemic consists of chronic diseases caused by unhealthy lifestyle choices. As adults, we must adopt these healthier lifestyle choices and show our children *by example* how to live healthier, happier lives.

According to emerging medical literature, we are on the brink of understanding epigenetics, a completely new aspect of biology that connects us to future generations in ways we never could have imagined. Epigenetics literally means "around the gene" and refers to the signals that instruct the gene how to behave.

According to this emerging science, not only do our genes receive instructions from our environment, but they also receive signals from generational changes to our ancestors' cells.

What does this mean for families? Well, a person might look at their family tree and see that they had one or two relatives who smoked their whole lives and lived cancer-free to age ninety-nine. You might infer that these people had "strong genes," and I would agree with you. However, any damage to their epigenetic code from smoking they did before having children will be passed on to the next generation. This does not change the gene itself but does make the next generation more susceptible to certain diseases, like cancer, as a result. For example, Dr. Michael Skinner, a professor at the School of Biological Sciences at Washington State University, says that if one of your grandparents is exposed to environmental toxins such as cigarette smoke or pesticides, you might be susceptible to disease even though you've never been exposed to the toxin. What's more, you will likely pass it on to your children and their descendants.[55]

Dr. Jonathan Seckl, Professor of Molecular Medicine Endocrinology Unit, Centre for Cardiovascular Science, Queen's Medical Research Institute University of Edinburgh, theorizes that it's not just genes but also the environmental impact from the early life of your ancestors. It's not so much "you are what you eat" as it's that you are what your mother ate and possibly what your grandmother ate. Following this line of thinking then, you are what *stresses* your grandmother or grandfather experienced, too.

Another way to look at the concept of genetics and epigenetics is this: Genes—our instructions—tell our bodies how to respond to particular cues from the environment. The genes themselves do not decide how to respond; they allow the body to respond exactly the way the instructions say to. As stated by Andrew Olaharski, Associate Director of Toxicology at Agios Pharmaceuticals, "Any type of toxicant in the environment that interacts with [epigenetic processes] can affect disease outcome."[56] While we all have the same basic set of genetic instructions, our sensitivities or predispositions to certain diseases can be passed down through the generations. For example, cancer runs in families. This means there may be a genetic weakness that predisposes the family members to cancer.

Despite this predisposition, 75 to 90 percent of cancers are environmentally caused, meaning a gene can only get "turned on" if the environmental trigger is present.[57] So if a predisposed person does not overexpose their body to environmental triggers, cancer may *not* likely be in their future. If 75 to 90 percent of all chronic illnesses, including cancers, are lifestyle-based, then we still have a great deal of control over the occurrence of the disease. According to Andrew Feinberg, MD, "We're not contradicting the view that genetic changes occur in the development of cancers, but there also are epigenetic changes and those come first." The gene and predisposition for cancer may exist, but it requires the right *signal* from an unhealthy environment for the gene to be activated.

Likewise, someone else may not be predisposed to cancer. Not one member of their family has ever had cancer. If their lifestyle is high in stress, sugar, and other toxins and they are sedentary most of the time, cancer may still be a possibility in their future. They are not immune to the disease just because they are not predisposed.

The reverse is also true. By living a healthy lifestyle, by feeding yourself everything that your body needs and not overexposing yourself to toxins, these epigenetic cues can be shut off just as easily as they can be turned on.

When it comes to our children, we must remember that they do not have a high capacity for decision making, especially when it comes to their health. I am sure 99 percent or more of children, if asked, would prefer ice cream, candy, soda, and hot dogs to fruits and vegetables. It is our responsibility as adults and parents to teach them these skills.

The best gift you can offer your children is to be a role model for good health. Show them what and how much to eat, how to live an active life, how to participate socially, and how to contribute to the economy. Children do not understand the consequences of their decisions, and allowing them to have whatever they want because it makes your life easier is only perpetuating the problem and significantly shortening their life span and their quality of life. We must all take responsibility for the health and well-being of our children and reverse current trends in their health. By doing so we can also start reversing these epigenetic codes in our families.

The current generation of children may be the first generation projected to die before their parents. That's pretty scary—and pathetic—especially since we know exactly why it is happening and exactly how to stop it from continuing.[58] There are absolutely no excuses! What's interesting is this comes at a time of a significant increase in life expectancy. Right now one of the fastest-growing populations is that of people living one hundred years or more. So, in just three generations, we will have gone from having the longest average life expectancy ever recorded to witnessing the first generation that may die younger than their parents did. We must learn to take responsibility for our health and the health of future generations right now.

CHAPTER TWELVE

YOU CAN TAKE RESPONSIBILITY FOR YOUR HEALTH RIGHT NOW

—

I hope you are now inspired to make some changes. Although improving your health may not always feel easy, once worked into your routine it *will* be very rewarding. You can expect to have a better quality of life, improved relationships, more energy, less stress, and more restful sleep. These changes will lead to other improvements as a ripple effect in multiple areas of your life.

Lifestyle change is not an all-or-nothing phenomenon. Chances are you will not wake up tomorrow with all your daily habits changed. This is okay! The purpose of this book is to give you options and choices to improve your health. Take a look at what you are willing to work on and start there.

Once you are comfortable with the changes—with your new lifestyle—your perception of health will be different and you can evaluate yourself again. You may be ready to incorporate a few more changes. The idea is to go slowly and remain comfortable. If you feel stress from the changes, it will be hard for you to maintain them. Just remember every healthy choice brings you closer to the wellness side of the continuum. Get there one choice at a time. If there is a sign of setback, do not beat yourself up about it. Love and forgive yourself enough to try again and get back on track. Most likely you will have a few bad days along the way. Expect it and enjoy the journey.

When I work with patients, I tailor a program similar to the one presented in this book, but I also include accountability. Accountability is key. When you know someone is watching and expecting your best performance, it helps keep you on track. This is human nature. Whether you can get to our office or not, find someone or work with someone who can hold you accountable. If you are making these changes as a family, hold each other accountable for the changes. This will dramatically improve your results.

Whether you choose to partner up or go it alone, follow these guidelines:

Know what you want, and set your goals specifically. Decide what vision you have in mind for your health. Do not focus on symptoms like weight, blood pressure, pain, or body fat. Focus on function—energy levels, bathroom habits, the ability to sit for long periods of time, and your emotional state of mind.

Make sure that your *choices* are congruent with your *goals*. If you are not sure what to focus on, how to develop a program, and/or whether your choices line up with your goals, find someone with the skills to help you. Everyone needs help on some level. Do not be too proud to ask for the help you need. It can only streamline your success. Good luck and enjoy the journey!

AFTERWORD

As far back as high school, I knew I wanted to be involed in health care. I felt a deep desire to help people improve their health. As a teenager I could see that it seemed we were, as a society, heading down an unhealthy path. I thought exercise would be my tool of choice so I could play my part in the health care solution, educating people on the importance of moving their bodies and motivating them to stay with it. After all, we already know how important exercise is for our health; the real challenge for people is starting a program and sticking to it. So I went to college, studied exercise science, and worked as a personal trainer for many years.

I quickly began to realize there are whole populations of people out there unable to exercise because they have other health problems that literally prevent them from moving their bodies. Post-surgical consequences, pain, chronic disease, loss of range of motion, or some other condition prevented them from exercising at a level that improved their health. That was how I got involved with chiropractic care.

I knew of chiropractic's value because years before, chiropractic care helped me heal from a wrestling injury in high school. I decided the knowledge and skills of a chiropractor combined with my background in exercise science would allow me to help people with chronic issues get to a place where they could begin an exercise program. Then I'd transition them from my care to an exercise professional who would develop exercise routines for them.

While studying to become a chiropractor, I learned about nutrition, stress management, pain management, exercise prescription, and rehabilitation. I never realized that chiropractic care could help so many people in such a variety of ways. I left school with myriad tools in my toolbox, ready to serve my patients.

In my own practice, I began seeing injured and infirm patients through a course of care that would prepare their bodies for daily activity by introducing chiropractic treatments, better nutrition, and proper exercise. Through my education and clinical experience, I realized there was another, much larger, population who needed my services just as much as the injured and unhealthy folks did. These people *thought* they were healthy; they generally had no symptoms of disease, but their health was slowly declining year after year. They were less able to participate in the activities and exercises they enjoyed, and they were being robbed of their ability to experience a high quality of life. You may be able to relate to this description as it describes the majority of Americans.

Some of you reading this book are active, while others of you may be sedentary. Often you find that you are uncomfortable enough to complain about some minor aches and pains, but not in enough pain to actually seek out the help of a doctor. You might experience some limited motion in your shoulders, back, knees, or hips but, again, not enough to go seek help. You might be a "weekend warrior" who is super active over the weekend (just enough to throw out an arm, strain a hamstring, or pull out your lower back) but get just enough rest to "recover" during the week in order to do it all over again the following weekend. Generally, the most common thought process is, "Why go to a doctor? What are they going to be able to do for me? Last time, he didn't even look at my complaint and wrote me a prescription for the pain and told me I was too old to perform that activity."

People who fit the above description, in my experience, are ticking time bombs. They were getting signals from their body for weeks, months, in some cases years, and either ignored them or did not know what to do or whom to see for help. They may eventually end up in our office or one like it when the big injury finally hits them. I would venture to say that at least 80 percent of them would never have needed us for this "crisis management" of a major injury if we were working with them months and years earlier when we could have helped them improve their body's performance along the way and regain muscular balance for injury prevention. All the subtle aches and pains over the years are a warning sign that your body is not functioning as well as it should. No, it's not just because you are getting older. There is no logical reason to live and put up with these issues. If these complaints are addressed properly over time, you should see an improvement in your ability to participate in life with less pain, more flexibility, and improved performance.

Some people do not know what chiropractic care is, nor what chiropractors really do for patients. They may have a vague notion that it's about "spinal adjustments," but it's really about improving nerve activity, improving range of motion, and keeping the body moving properly to ensure the balance of our systems. Along with this focus, our goal is to minimize the chances of potential injuries. This is accomplished through spinal adjustments, as well as muscle work, exercises, and nutritional counseling. Think of chiropractors as the maintenance crew for your body.

I find that everyone has their own rhythms and needs when it comes to their treatment. As discussed earlier, it all depends on the amount and type of stress you have in your life, your diet, and exercise routines. Personally, I see a chiropractor once or twice a month. This rhythm allows me the freedom to work hard, exercise with intensity, and play hard without worrying that any old injuries are going to sneak up on me. That's what chiropractic care is all about. I am an avid rock climber, I exercise vigorously during the week, I like to go camping and hiking, and enjoy playing with my children. Taking care of myself this way allows me to pursue all the activities that give me pleasure in my life. It helps me maintain the high quality of life I desire and demand.

There are many versions of how chiropractic care is actually practiced. Regardless of the exact type of treatment, the goals and outcomes are the same: to improve the body's ability to perform. I urge you to find a local chiropractor and have an evaluation. If you've seen one before and were not happy with your care, find another one. Just like if you had an experience with a dentist you were not pleased with, you wouldn't say, "Dentistry just didn't work for me." You would find another dentist, because your oral health is important. Equally important is using chiropractic care for the maintenance of your physical health. Try a few offices until you find the right practitioner for you.

BE FIT EXERCISES

~

THE SEVEN-DAY FITNESS PROGRAM

I have designed an exercise schedule based on seven workout days per week. Seven days of exercise may sound like a lot, but the program is structured with varying intensity and duration per day. Some days the exercises may take you five or ten minutes to complete, while other days your workout may take a little more than an hour throughout the day.

Don't feel pressured to complete the elements all at once. You can complete your flexibility training in the morning and your strength training after lunch or in the evening if that works better for your schedule. You can even spread your strength exercises throughout the day (i.e. your push-ups can be done in increments of five or ten push-ups an hour until you have finished all your reps).

Begin your program on any day of the week, but keep track of the schedule once you begin. If you miss a workout day during the week, skip that day's workout and move on to the following day in the program. Each day of the week, be sure to include five to ten minutes of flexibility and range of motion work. Without this component, you will be vulnerable to injury, limited in your ability to participate in daily activities, and you will be starving your brain and nerves of the information it needs regarding the limits of your body and understanding of how it moves. Physical movement provides our brain with information crucial for body awareness and proper function. Without proper movement and flexibility we become deficient in this information, therefore "starving" ourselves of neuromuscular health.

SEVEN-DAY FITNESS PROGRAM

Day 1	Day 2	Day 3	Day 4	Day 5	Day 6	Day 7
Flexibility 5–10 min	Flexibility 5–10 min	Flexibility 5–10 min	Flexibility 5–10 min	Flexibility 5–10 min	Flexibility 5–10 min	Flexibility 5–10 min
High Intensity 5–8 min	Endurance 30–60 min	High Intensity 5–8 min	Endurance 30–60 min	Intervals 20–45 min	Endurance 30–60 min	Recovery
Strength 1 to approx. 30 min		Strength 1 to approx. 30 min		Strength 2 to approx. 20 min		

I've prescribed three strength days, three endurance days, two high-intensity days, and one day of interval training, because the human body should move in different ways and in different intensities every day. The days are spaced and combined in a way that maximizes the effectiveness and efficiency of time spent exercising, as well as to limit the chances of injury. Although at first glance it may look like a lot of work and a large time commitment, with familiarity you will see that this program becomes quite manageable and fairly easy to maintain. Once you have exhausted the benefits of my

Be Fit program, I encourage you to look for exercise outlets. You could join a gym, hire a personal trainer, or find a boot camp to participate in. At some point you will need further instruction in order to set new goals and continue improving your fitness.

Flexibility Workouts

The flexibility training outlined below is an essential component of the seven-day fitness program. Perform each exercise every day. Once you get the hang of each movement, you will only need to spend five to ten minutes per day to complete this portion of the workout. If you are new to exercise or especially out of shape, you may want to focus solely on this part of the workout for a few weeks before incorporating the rest of the program components.

- **Spinal Flexibility**: You must take care of your spine if you want to keep it intact and free of injury. Improving spinal mobility requires you to work your spine's full range of motion everyday by including flexion/extension, rotation, and lateral bending to the right and left. Hold each of these positions for ten to twelve seconds before moving to the next position. Complete two sets of each movement. Range of motion exercises should be performed for your neck, as well as your mid- and lower-back.

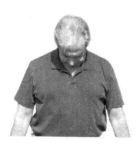

Neck flexion forward, touching chin to chest.

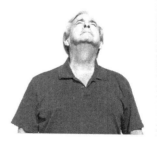

Neck extension, reaching chin to sky.

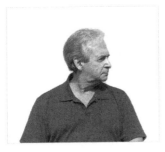

Neck rotation, turning chin to the left.

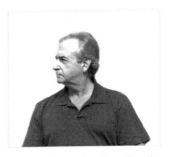

Neck rotation, turning chin to the right.

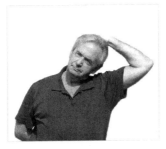

Lateral flexion to the left.

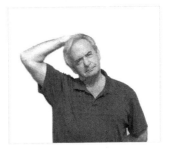

Lateral flexion to the right.

- **YTWL exercises**: So many of the very common rotator cuff injuries are due to a lack of muscular support in the shoulders. Proper movement and contraction of your shoulder blades will protect your rotator cuff from overuse injuries. YTWL exercises are an easy and effective way to improve

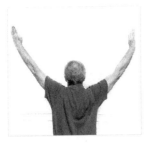

Make a Y with your arms raised above your head.

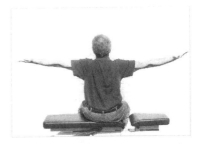

Extend your arms outward to make a T.

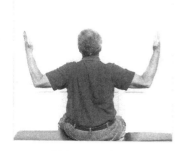

*Make a W with your
arms at your sides.*

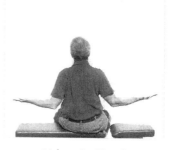

*Make an L with each
arm at your sides.*

the scapular strength and coordination you want to maintain healthy shoulders. You should be squeezing your shoulder blades together during each pose. Hold each arm position for a count of fifteen seconds before moving to the next position. Complete two sets.

- **Squats (Wall Sit/Full Squat):** Squatting requires flexibility and stability in the hips, back, shoulders, and ankles. It is also good practice for some of the other exercises in this program. Once in the squat position, or as far into the

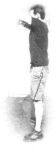

*Begin your squat in standing position,
with your hands pressed together in
front of your breastbone.*

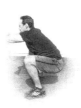

*Squat down as far as possible, keeping
your hands in place.*

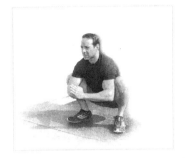 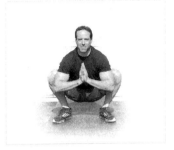

Hold your squat for twenty to thirty seconds. You can also press your elbows into the inside of your knees for a deeper hip stretch.

position as you are comfortable, hold the pose for twenty to thirty seconds and then stand up. Complete two sets.

- **Pigeon**: This is a great stretch for the glutes and hip muscles. Balance of tension between the hips, glutes, and hip flexors is paramount to preventing injury of the lower back and hips.

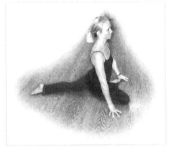 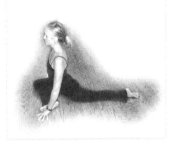

Active pigeon stretch, from the right.   *Active pigeon stretch, from the left.*

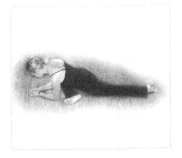

Passive pigeon stretch. Slowly bend forward over your bent knee. Bend only as far as to feel a light stretch in your back and hips.

There are two ways to do this; I recommend both the active and passive versions. Hold each pose for thirty seconds

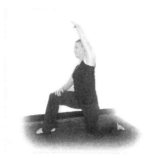

Kneel in a lunging position. Raise the arm opposite your lunging leg and reach over your head until you feel a stretch. Repeat on the opposite side.

before switching to the other leg.

- **Hip Flexor-Wall**: It's essential to maintain balance in the complex muscles around the hips and spine. Tight hip flexors are one of the most common causes of lower back failure and injury. We get this tightness primarily from sitting all the time. Hold the pose for thirty seconds on each side.

- **Foam Roll**: This simple but effective tool is a great aid in working out the kinks from the day and for preparing your muscles for a workout. I recommend doing a quick, full body roll once or twice per day to address all the major muscle

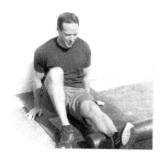

Technique for foam rolling the calf. Repeat on opposite leg.

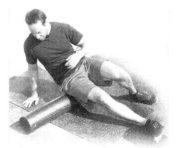

Technique for foam rolling the glute. Repeat on opposite glute.

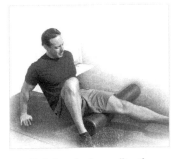

Technique for foam rolling the hamstring. Repeat on opposite leg.

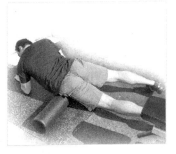

Technique for foam rolling the hip flexor. Repeat on opposite leg.

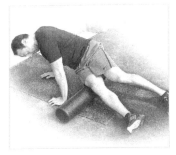

Technique for foam rolling the IT band. Repeat on opposite leg.

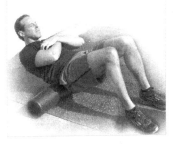

Technique for foam rolling the lower back.

groups. For example, roll before starting your exercise routine, and roll again at the end of the day to relax and open the muscles that have been used too much or not enough in your daily activities. The whole process should take about three to four minutes.

High-Intensity Endurance Workouts

Day 1 and Day 3 include a high-intensity endurance workout and a strength workout. The high-intensity workouts are all-out, 100 percent efforts for short bursts of time. Most of them will take a total of five or six minutes to complete. You can plug in any of the exercises listed below for your high-intensity days. You will likely prefer certain exercises to others, but I encourage you to vary your choice of workout each time for the best results. Although short, these exercises are intense and you should feel tired after they are completed. As your fitness improves, so will your speed. When first starting out just push yourself to complete the exercises. As you progress, push yourself to beat previous speeds, times, or repetitions.

Choose one of the following exercises per session:

- **Jump Rope**: 30 seconds jumping, 30 seconds rest **or** 100 jumps on, 30 seconds rest. Repeat for five minutes.

- **Sprint**: 50-meter dash, 30-second rest. Repeat five times, then 100-meter dash, 60-second rest. Repeat five times.

- **Row**: 100 to 250–meter row, 90 seconds rest. Repeat five times.

- **Burpees**: 30 seconds on, 30 seconds rest. Repeat three times, then 45 seconds on, 90 seconds rest. Repeat two times.

- **Swim:** 100-meter sprint, then two minutes rest. Repeat three times. Then, 50-meter sprint, thirty seconds rest. Repeat five times.

- **Bike:** Half-mile sprint, sixty seconds relaxed pace. Repeat eight times.

Low-Intensity Endurance Workouts

These endurance workouts are low-intensity, longer-duration workouts. They will take you somewhere between thirty and sixty minutes but should be completed at a pace and intensity that allows you to talk and feel relatively comfortable during the workouts. If you are breathing too heavily to maintain a conversation, you are working too hard! Low-intensity endurance workouts can be chosen from the list of recommendations on the following pages, or you can program your own. Try to incorporate different cardiovascular exercises each day you do your endurance workouts, or at least keep changing between two or three different types.

A comfortable pace will be around 55 to 75 percent of your maximum heart rate (MHR). To calculate your MHR, follow this equation: MHR = 220 − (your age). Then, to establish your comfortable pace, multiply that number by .55 and again by .75. For example, a fifty-five-year-old would have a heart rate of somewhere between 91–124 during endurance exercise routines.

Choose one of the following exercises per session:

- Walk: 2–5 miles
- Run: 2–6 miles
- Hike: 2–5 miles
- Row: 4–8 miles
- Swim: 1–2 miles
- Golf: 9–18 holes (walking the course)
- Bike: 8–20 miles
- Gardening: 30–60 minutes
- Yard Work: 30–60 minutes
- House Cleaning: 30–60 minutes

Interval Workouts

An interval workout will have a varied pace, incorporating high- and moderate-intensity movements. This will train your body to change gears rapidly, increase blood flow and oxygen levels, and encourage quick recovery from short bursts of fast movements.

Choose one workout for your Day 5 session:

- **Run**: 400 meters at an easy jog, then sprint for 200 meters. Repeat six to eight times.

- **Row**: 500 meters at an easy pace, then sprint for 100 meters. Repeat six to eight times.

- **Swim**: freestyle or breaststroke 150 meters at an easy pace (six lengths or three laps in most pools), then swim very quickly for 100 meters (four lengths or two laps). Repeat six to eight times.

- **Bike**: one mile at an easy pedal, then pedal hard for a quarter-mile sprint. Repeat six to eight times.

Strength Workouts

The strength portion of your workout will take somewhere between twenty to forty minutes to complete when you first start the program. Once you are familiar with the movements, it should take twenty minutes or less. There are many great strength programs out there. Some require the heavy equipment that you would find at a commercial gym. Some require very little or no equipment. Generally I find that exercises that utilize your body weight are the most beneficial and help you prepare your body for the tasks of life. So, for the purposes of this program, I propose five basic, full-body movements (push-ups, pull-ups, squats, planks, and overhead press) that require minimal equipment (a pull-up bar, a pair of dumbbells, and exercise bands) that can be purchased at the sporting goods store. You can complete these movements at home or in a gym.

HOW TO ASSESS YOUR CURRENT STRENGTH

It is important to place yourself in the proper progression level for each exercise. To determine where you should begin with your strength training, you must try each movement and determine your strength level with every exercise. Based upon the assessment, you can clearly determine where your strength workouts should start and how you should progress through the series of exercises. It is common to be at different progression levels for different exercises. For example, you may find that you have a stronger lower body than upper body. This is perfectly normal and not unexpected.

The assessment is simple; try each movement on the exercise list. Allow yourself an hour to complete it. Start with the standard version of each movement. The standard, mid-range version is called "Progression 4" and is marked with a double asterisk. If you can do at least the minimum amount of the exercise listed, then you are working at the correct level. If you cannot do the minimum amount listed, try the less-intense version of that movement. If you try the exercise and can already do the maximum amount, move forward and try a harder version of that exercise.

Let's use push-ups as an example:

	Minimum Reps	Maximum Reps
Progression 1: Wall push-up	5	75
Progression 2: Incline/bench push-up	5	75
Progression 3: Knee push-up	5	75
** Progression 4: Traditional push-up	5	75
Progression 5: Hand-release push-up	5	75
Progression 6: Decline push-up	5	75

Progression 4 for this exercise has a minimum of five push-ups. If you can do five push-ups right now, then Progression 4 is the correct exercise level for you. In that case you would execute seventy-five push-ups on your strength day, which could be done in three sets of twenty-five, five to seven sets of ten to twelve reps with a minute rest in between, or as many sets of five as you can do throughout the day until you reach your target of seventy-five push-ups. Ultimately, it is best to try to get them done in as short a period of time as possible but, especially in the early stages of your strength training, it is fine to spread them out.

If you cannot do five push-ups in a row, you try Progression 3. If you can do five knee push-ups, then you would stick with knee push-ups until you can move up to regular push-ups. If knee push-ups are too difficult, move to Progression 2 or even Progression 1 (incline push-ups and wall push-ups, respectively) until you find a comfortable place to begin. If seventy-five regular push-ups are already attainable, move up to Progressions 5, or 6, until you reach a challenging level. It is essential to know what level is appropriate for your strength level before you really push yourself. Follow the progression assessment with each exercise so that you identify the level at which you should begin each exercise.

This self-assessment is used to determine which progression of the exercises you should be using for your Strength 1 Workouts (Days 1 and 3). As you reach each progression's maximum reps comfortably, you will move to the next exercise progression. On your Strength 2 Workouts (Day 5), you will begin to introduce that next progression of exercise. In the example from above, if you are able to do seventy-five wall push-ups, you should move to incline/bench push-ups for Strength 1 Workout day. You will stay with incline push-ups until seventy-five reps become attainable. On your Strength 2 Workout day you will attempt knee push-ups (which is the next progression). When you are trying the harder version of the exercises, try only one to ten repetitions at the most.

This Day 2 strength workout is not meant to push your strength limits as much as it meant is to introduce your body to new modifications of the exercise and to prepare you for your next progression. On these days, just a few reps are more than enough. If you cannot yet do one full rep, even getting in the proper position for the movement and preparing to do it may be enough for this day. Therefore your Strength 2 Workout may be shorter in time from your Strength 1 day.

Strength 1 Workouts: Develop strength within your particular transitional program based on your assessment test and progress.

Strength 2 Workouts: Challenge yourself with trying one to ten repetitions ("reps") of each exercise, one progression more advanced than what you are currently doing.

STRENGTH WORKOUT PROGRESSIONS

Push-up

	Minimum Reps	Maximum Reps
Progression 1: Wall push-up	5	75
Progression 2: Incline/bench push-up	5	75
Progression 3: Knee push-up	5	75
** Progression 4: Traditional push-up	5	75
Progression 5: Hand-release push-up	5	75
Progression 6: Decline push-up	5	75

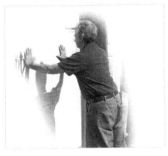 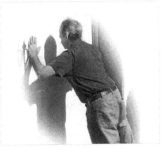

Progression 1: A wall, or standing, push-up uses a vertical surface for support, facilitating someone who cannot bear their full weight on their upper body, knees, and toes.

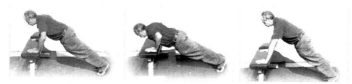

Progression 2: An incline push-up, using a bench for support of the upper body.

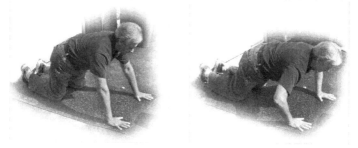

*Progression 3: A knee push up, with knees and toes on the mat,
lessens the amount of weight the arms must lift.*

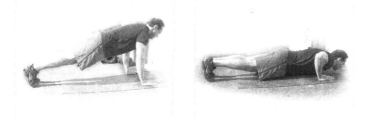

Progression 4: A traditional push-up, with the body parallel to the mat.

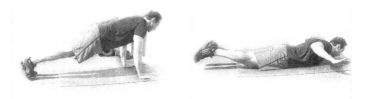

*Progression 5: In a hand-release push-up the weight is released from the
hands with each repetition before pushing back up to the starting position.*

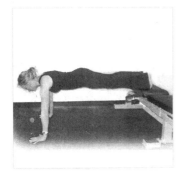 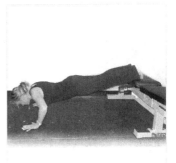

*Progression 6: A decline push-up, with feet supported on a bench,
increases the difficulty of the exercise.*

Knees to Elbows

	Minimum Reps	Maximum Reps
Progression 1: Practice hanging	2 sets of 3 reps of 30 seconds to 1 minute	—
Progression 2: Knee lifts to 45 degrees	5	25
Progression 3: Knee lifts to 90 degrees	5	25
**Progression 4: Knee to elbow	5	25
Progression 5: Toes to bar	5	25

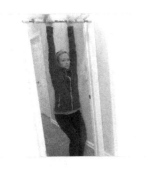 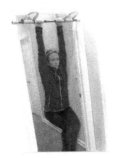

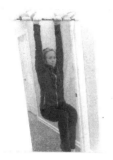 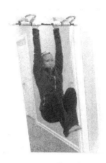

Progressions 1–4: Begin with your hands grasping a pull-up bar and your legs in neutral. Depending on your strength, complete repetitions by lifting your knees to 45 degrees, 90 degrees, or all the way to your elbows. As your strength increases try more challenging lifts.

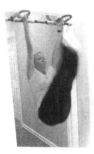 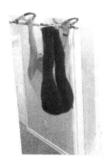

Progression 5: For a greater challenge, try lifting your toes to the bar.

Squat

	Minimum Reps	Maximum Reps
Progression 1: Wall sit	0–10 seconds	60 seconds
Progression 2: Ball squat	5 reps	75 reps
Progression 3: Air squat	5 reps	75 reps
** Progression 4: Weighted squat	5 reps	10–50 reps
Progression 5: Squat thrust*	5 reps	10–50 reps

*The squat thrust is the combination of two separate movements, the squat and the overhead press, into one complex and fluid movement.

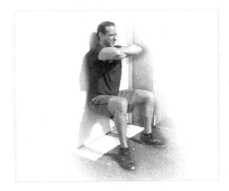

*Progression 1: A wall-sit is a variation on the squat, focusing on the quadriceps.
Place your back against a flat, vertical surface and your feet and knees hip-distance
apart. Gradually move into a sitting position, keeping your knees bent at right angles.*

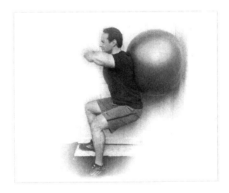

*Progression 2: With an inflatable exercise ball between your back
and the wall, execute a full squat using the ball for support.*

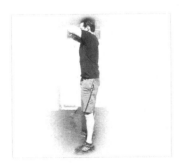
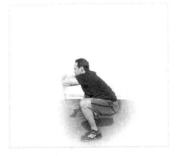

*Progression 3: From standing position with your feet wider than hip-distance, squat
down. You may only be able to squat to about 90 degrees initially, but eventually
your hips should extend below the level of your knees.*

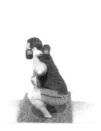 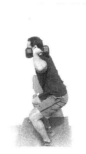

Progression 4: A variation on the traditional squat is to use hand weights to increase the strength required to complete the movement.

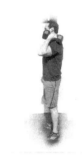 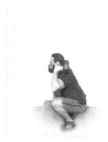 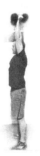

Progression 5: A squat thrust is a modified squat in which you will thrust upward with more power and quickness than in the traditional, weighted squat, and then fully extend your arms at the top of the movement.

Plank

	Minimum Reps	Maximum Reps
Progression 1: Hands and knees	0–45 seconds	1 minute/2 sets
Progression 2: Hands and toes	1–45 seconds	1 minute/2 sets
Progression 3: Elbows and knees	1–45 seconds	1 minute/2 sets
**Progression 4: Elbows and toes (plank)	1–45 seconds	1 minute/2 sets
Progression 5: Side plank	1–45 seconds	1 minute/2 sets

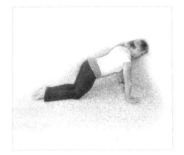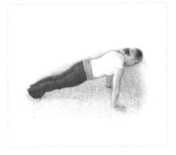

Progression 1 and 2: A straight-arm plank may be
done with bent knees or straight legs.

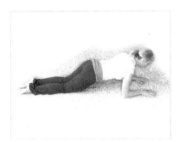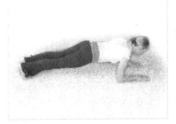

Progression 3 and 4: A bent-arm plank, with forearms on the mat,
may be done with bent knees or straight legs.

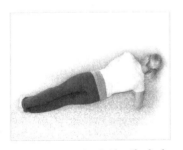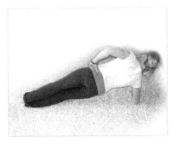

Progression 5: The side plank may be done with one arm extended
out to support the body or with the free arm resting on the hip.

Overhead Press

	Minimum Reps	Maximum Reps
Progression 1: Overhead stretch	full range of motion overhead	20, no weight
Progression 2: Light press	5, 5–10-pound press	40, 5–10-pound press
Progression 3: Moderate press	5, 15–25-pound press	40, 15–25-pound press
** Progression 4: Heavy press	5, 30–45-pound press	40, 30–45-pound press

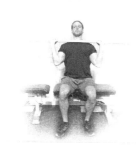 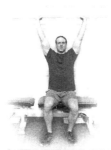

Progression 1: In a seated position, with a weight bar, broomstick, or length of PVC pipe, extend your arms from collarbone to the ceiling.

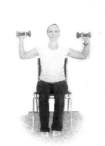 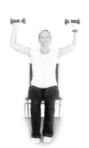 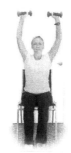

Progressions 2–4: In a seated position, using dumbbells, begin with your arms at 90 degree angles. Extend your arms upward until the dumbbells are a little closer than shoulder-width apart. Increase the weight of your dumbbells as needed.

Pull-up

	Minimum Reps	Maximum Reps
Progression 1: Chair/pull-up	0–5	20
Progression 2: Jumping pull-up	2–6	20
Progression 3: Flexed-arm hang	10–60 seconds	2 sets of 60 seconds
** Progression 4: Pull-up	2–5	25

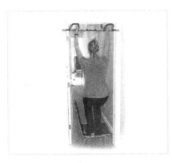 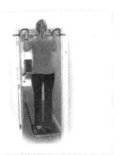

Progression 1: Standing on a chair with bent knees, stand up to the pull-up bar. This allows you to execute a pull-up without supporting your full body weight. Slowly try to increase the weight in your arms by decreasing the assistance of your legs in supporting you.

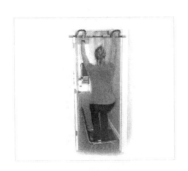 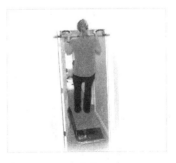

Progression 2: Standing on a chair, jump up to the bar. The momentum from jumping will help you reach the bar.

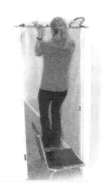

*Progression 3: For the flexed-arm hang,
hang from the pull-up bar with your arms bent.*

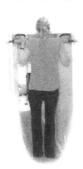

*Progression 4: In the traditional pull-up, hang from the bar
and pull yourself upwards until your chin is over the bar.*

BE NOURISHED RECIPES

~

Once you get the hang of my recommendations, food planning will be easy. The list of ingredients is simple: Fruits, vegetables, nuts, seeds, and meat are the basics of what to eat on a daily basis. Be mindful that your ingredients are not genetically modified (GMO) and don't contain added chemicals, preservatives, or pharmaceuticals. Keep your meals interesting by mixing up cooking styles, changing meal presentations, and trying new spices.

BREAKFAST SUGGESTIONS

1. A few (one to three) pasture-raised, hormone- and antibiotic-free eggs. These can be prepared numerous ways and with various additional ingredients, like potato, spinach, tomato, and leftover chicken or steak. Pretty much any healthy food on the list that you like can be added to your eggs. Get creative! Poached and over-easy are the healthiest preparations, but scrambled, over-medium, omelet style, or frittata are okay, too. Try not to overcook the eggs, as some nutrients are heat sensitive and may be destroyed by overcooking.

2. A healthy protein and/or fruit smoothie. Here are some guidelines to follow in composing your smoothie:

- You will need a liquid base. I recommend rice milk, almond milk, coconut milk, or even water. Be sure to choose unsweetened varieties to avoid adding unnecessary sugar. Try to avoid the ingredient carrageenan whenever possible. It is commonly found in many nut milks. If you can, consider making your own nut or rice milk.
- Add fresh or frozen organic fruit with no added sugar (berries are a great choice).
- If you have a powerful blender you can add some vegetables or a few ounces of organic vegetable juice.
- It is important to have some protein in the shake to facilitate absorption of the fat-soluble vitamins in the fruit and vegetables. This can come from nuts and seeds or organic nut butters like almond or cashew. Or you can use a protein powder. I recommend using a rice or pea (vegetable-based) protein instead of whey protein, which is a dairy by-product. If you must use protein powders, make sure they are derived from grass-fed cows.

I have included some of my favorite smoothie recipes for you to try.

Smoothie #1
1 ½ cups fresh spinach leaves
1 cup strawberries
½ cup blackberries or blueberries
2 cups coconut milk
5 ice cubes
Handful of walnuts or almonds
Blend and enjoy

Smoothie #2
1 cup frozen or fresh kale
1 cup raspberries
½ cup blackberries
1 banana

Handful of walnuts or almonds
2 cups coconut milk
Blend and enjoy

Smoothie #3
½ head of romaine lettuce
1 large organic carrot
½ ripe avocado (this will make the smoothie very creamy,
like a mousse)
½ cup raw spinach or kale
2 cups coconut milk
1 ½ cups frozen berries
5 ice cubes
Handful of walnuts or almonds
Blend and enjoy

Smoothie #4
1 cup water
Kale to fill blender cup
Protein powder of choice
Blend those together and then add:
Two bananas
Frozen peaches
Blend again and enjoy

Smoothie #5
1 cup almond milk
Handful of kale
Handful collard greens or spinach
One carrot
One apple
½ lemon
Vegetable-based protein powder of choice
Frozen peaches
Blend and enjoy

Smoothie #6

2 cups water
1 cup coconut water
3 handfuls kale
1 ½ banana
Frozen green grapes
Two kiwis
1 cup pineapple
Blend and enjoy

Smoothie #7

4 cups almond milk
Four dates
Two bananas
2 cups ice
½ teaspoon cinnamon
Vanilla protein powder
Blend and enjoy

Other Breakfast Ideas

Muffin Omelet

These are quick, easy, and great for a grab-and-go breakfast. Toddlers love them, too!

12 eggs
1 cup diced peppers or any vegetable of choice

Beat the eggs, mix in the peppers, pour into greased muffin tins. Bake at 400 degrees for twenty minutes.

Silver Dollar Pancakes

1 ½ cups almond or rice flour
1 ½ cups coconut milk
5 eggs
1 cup blueberries
1 teaspoon vanilla
1 teaspoon cinnamon

Heat skillet and coat with coconut oil. Mix all ingredients. Pour silver-dollar–sized portion of batter into skillet and let sit until bubbles form on the top. Then flip. Once both sides are golden brown, they're done. Serve with a little bit of maple syrup.

Sweet Potato Hash

2 tablespoons coconut oil
4 strips nitrate-free bacon, cut into small pieces
3 sweet potatoes, peeled and diced
¼ cup red onion, diced

Place coconut oil in pan over medium heat. Once melted, add bacon. After two minutes add sweet potatoes and onion and let sit until they begin to brown. Toss and brown the other side. Continue to stir occasionally until desired crispness of potatoes is achieved. Add salt or pepper to taste before serving.

Homemade Health Bars

Oatmeal Apple Breakfast Bars

Wet ingredients:
Two bananas
¼ cup applesauce
¼ cup pumpkin puree

Dry ingredients:
One apple, chopped
2 cups dry oats
2 tablespoons flax seed
½ cup raisins
½ cup raw nuts
Cinnamon, to taste

Mix banana, applesauce, and pumpkin in a blender and pour into a large mixing bowl. Combine apple, oats, and remaining dry ingredients. Add to the wet mixture. Fold gently with a spatula or wooden spoon. Bake in a 8"-by-8" baking dish at 350 degrees for twenty minutes. Cool and cut into squares for serving.

Cheryl Bars

These bars are very versatile, customized to your liking. You can substitute applesauce for the water, add ¼ cup of your preferred nut butter, add raw coconut flakes, etc. The more you play with it, the more you will make it your own.

1 cup pitted dates
1 cup raw nuts and/or seeds (almonds, cashews, sunflower seeds, and/or pumpkin seeds)
½ cup raisins and/or cran-raisins
1 tablespoon water

Combine everything in a food processor and puree until mixture starts to come together. Add a little water as necessary until mixture sticks together.

Take spoonfuls of the mixture and roll into balls. Place on cookie sheet to dry as cookies, or flatten in a baking pan and cut to make bars.

If they're a little too wet you can bake them at 225 degrees for about thirty minutes. For best results, store them in the refrigerator.

Sweet Potato Pineapple Muffins

Wet ingredients:

1 cup mashed, cooked sweet potato

4 egg whites

1 whole egg

1 teaspoon vanilla

Dry ingredients:

2 cups almond flour

½ teaspoon pumpkin pie spice

1 tablespoon baking powder

Fruit and nuts:

½ cup chopped pineapple

½ cup walnuts

½ cup raisins

Combine wet ingredients in a bowl. Mix dry ingredients in another bowl. Add dry mixture to wet mixture and stir. Add in pineapple, walnuts, and raisins. Spoon into muffin tins. Bake at 350 degrees for twenty-five minutes.

Lunch/Dinner Suggestions

1. Salad with grilled fish or chicken. The salad should contain mixed vegetables and a variety of colors. To ensure you're getting most or all the nutrients possible, try to use all the colors you can find. Use three to five cups of vegetables with three to four ounces of protein (a piece of meat about the size of your palm).

2. Grilled or steamed vegetables with a side of protein (i.e., chicken, fish, beef, or pork).

3. Hearty homemade vegetable and meat-based soups.

Lunch and Dinner Recipes

Spaghetti Squash Casserole
1 large spaghetti squash, halved lengthwise

1 pound ground beef

2 tablespoons olive oil

3 cloves garlic, chopped

3 cups spinach

1 (10-ounce) can crushed tomatoes

1 teaspoon red pepper flakes

1 teaspoon Italian seasoning

Heat oven to 350 degrees. Cook squash on a baking sheet with small amount of water for forty-five to fifty minutes or until tender. Shred with fork once cooled. Transfer cooked spaghetti squash to casserole dish and set aside. Leave oven on. Cook ground beef in skillet over medium heat until no longer pink. Drain and add to spaghetti squash. Add olive oil to skillet over medium heat. Add and sauté garlic until slightly browned. Add spinach and cook until wilted. Top spaghetti squash and meat with spinach/garlic mixture. Top with crushed tomatoes and seasoning. Return to oven for fifteen minutes to allow all ingredients to cook together. Serve warm.

Nut-crusted Chicken
2 tablespoons coconut oil

2 eggs

1 cup chopped pecans

1 cup chopped walnuts

4 chicken breasts

Warm coconut oil in skillet over medium heat. Scramble eggs in bowl. Place chopped nuts in separate bowl. Dip chicken breasts in egg mixture, then nut mixture, then add to skillet. Cook until browned and chicken is cooked through.

Chicken Fajitas
4 (4-ounce) uncooked chicken breasts
1 tablespoon olive oil
1 sliced onion
1 green bell pepper, sliced into strips
1 red bell pepper, sliced into strips
lime wedges for serving

Season chicken breasts with your choice of spices (garlic powder, cumin, chili powder, salt, pepper, etc.) and marinate in a resealable bag for an hour. Heat the oil in a skillet over high heat. Add onion, peppers, and chicken to the skillet, stirring occasionally until vegetables are just tender and the chicken is cooked through, about ten minutes. Transfer to serving dish and enjoy with lime wedges.

Quinoa and Cranberries Salad
3 cups dry quinoa, cooked and cooled
1 cup dried cranberries
1 cup sliced almonds
Scallions sliced very thin, both white and green parts (amount to be adjusted according to personal taste)
1 can mandarin oranges, drained

Dressing:
⅓ cup orange juice
¼ olive oil
Orange rind, grated

Combine all ingredients and serve at room temp.

Black Rice and Sweet Potatoes

1 cup black rice
2 cups water or broth
2 tablespoons olive oil
1 ½ cup scallions, chopped
2 tablespoons peeled, minced fresh ginger
½ diced red bell pepper
2 sweet potatoes, peeled, and cut into ½-inch cubes
Season to taste with salt, black pepper, and/or cayenne pepper

Bring rice, water, and dash of salt to a boil in a pot. Reduce heat to low and cook rice, covered, until most of water is absorbed, about twenty minutes. While rice cooks, heat oil in a large skillet over medium-high heat and sauté scallions, ginger, red pepper, and sweet potatoes. Cover and cook, stirring occasionally, until potatoes are just tender, about fifteen minutes. Add rice and toss gently to combine. Season to taste.

Black Bean Salad

1 diced avocado
2 cans black beans, drained and rinsed (16-ounce cans)
1 diced tomato
1 bunch chopped fresh parsley
1 red onion, diced

Dressing:
¼ cup balsamic vinegar
2 tablespoons olive oil
1 teaspoon lemon juice
1 teaspoon minced garlic
1 teaspoon honey
Salt
Ground black pepper

Lettuce leaves

In a large bowl, combine the avocado, beans, tomato, parsley, and onion. Mix the vinegar, oil, lemon juice, garlic, and honey and add to bean mixture. Let the salad marinate for thirty minutes at room temperature. Add salt and pepper to taste. Arrange lettuce leaves on four salad plates; spoon salad over the lettuce.

Butternut Squash Soup

2 stalks celery, diced
1 onion, diced
2 tablespoons olive oil
32 ounces stock, chicken or vegetable
2 potatoes, diced
2 carrots, diced
1 large butternut squash, peeled, cubed, and seeded
salt and pepper to taste

Sauté celery and onions in oil for five minutes. Add gluten-free stock, potatoes, carrots, and squash. Simmer forty-five minutes. When everything is softened, puree in a blender until smooth. Season to taste.

You might also add a 10-ounce package of spinach instead of the squash to make a delicious spinach soup.

Split Pea Soup

1 pound split peas
3 quarts water
1 diced onion
4 diced carrots
4 diced celery stalks
¼ bunch parsley
¼ bunch dill
3 cloves garlic
½ teaspoon cumin
1 teaspoon each salt and pepper

Combine all ingredients in a large pot and after it comes to a boil, lower to a simmer and cook for about three hours covered.

Snack Ideas

1. Trail mix (raw nuts and seeds with a little dried fruit)
2. Celery or apple with nut butter (sunflower butter, almond butter, or cashew butter)
3. Powdered vegetable/fruit drink (There are numerous freeze-dried and powdered fruit and vegetable drinks available. They are very healthy to consume and easy to make—just a scoop of powder and add water. They are great when you need to grab something and just run out of the house.)
4. Smoothie (see recipes)
5. Homemade health bars (see recipes)
6. Avocado with oil and lemon
7. Hummus with veggies

NUTRITION BOOKS

I have found the following books to be very informative and helpful in learning about a healthy diet and for identifying new recipes to incorporate into your diet.

The Paleo Diet: Lose Weight and Get Healthy by Eating the Food You Were Designed to Eat, revised edition by Loren Cordain

The Paleo Solution: The Original Human Diet by Robb Wolf

In Defense of Food: An Eater's Manifesto by Michael Pollan

The Big Book of Health and Fitness: A Practical Guide to Diet, Exercise, Healthy Aging, Illness Prevention, and Sexual Well-Being by Philip Maffeton

Eat Fat, Lose Fat: Lose Weight And Feel Great With The Delicious, Science-based Coconut Diet by Sally Fallon and Mary Enig

Wheat Belly: Lose the Wheat, Lose the Weight, and Find Your Path Back to Health by William Davis, MD

The Omnivore's Dilemma: A Natural History of Four Meals by Michael Pollan

The Whole Life Nutrition Cookbook: Whole Foods Recipes for Personal and Planetary Health, second edition, by Alissa Segersten and Tom Malterre

Nourishing Traditions: The Cookbook that Challenges Politically Correct Nutrition and the Diet Dictocrats by Sally Fallon

NOTES

1   Hsiang-Ching Kung, PhD, et al., "Deaths: Final Data for 2005," *National Vital Statistics Reports* 56, no. 10 (2008), http://www.cdc.gov/nchs/data/nvsr/nvsr56/nvsr56_10.pdf.

2   Ibid.

3   Linda L.Barrett, PhD, "Prescription Drug Use Among Midlife and Older Americans," *AARP Study* (January 2005), http://www.aarp.org/health/drugs-supplements/info-2005/rx_midlife_plus.html.

4   Ibid.

5   Ibid.

6   American Chemical Society, "Record 4.12 Billion Prescriptions in the United States in 2011," *Medical News Today*, (September 14, 2012), http://www.medicalnewstoday.com/releases/250213.php.

7   Scott K. Powers and Edward T. Howley, *Exercise Physiology*, 3rd ed. (New York: McGraw-Hill, 1997), 17–19.

8   Charles R. Scriver, et al., eds., *The Metabolic and Molecular Bases of Inherited Disease*, 7th ed. (New York: McGraw-Hill, Health Professions Division, 1995).

9   SB Eaton, et al., "Evolutionary Health Promotion," *Preventative Medicine* 34 (2002): 109–118.

10 Ibid.

11 Amy Ralston, PhD, and Kenna Shaw, PhD, "Environment Controls Gene Expression: Sex Determination and the Onset of Genetic Disorders," *Nature Education* 1, no.1 (2008); Ingrid Lobo, "Environmental Influences on Gene Expression," *Nature Education 1*, no. 1 (2008); Anura Hewagama and Bruce Richardson, "The Genetics and Epigenetics of Autoimmune Diseases," *Journal of Autoimmunity* 33 no.1 (August 2009): 3–11, doi:10.1016/jaut.2009.03.007; Keith M Godfrey, et al., "Epigenetic Gene Promoter Methylation at Birth Is Associated with Child's Later Adiposity," *Diabetes* 60, no. 5 (May 2011): 1528-34, doi:102337/db 10-0979; Thea M. Edwards and John Peterson Myers, "Environmental Exposures and Gene Regulation in Disease Etiology,"

Environmental Health Perspectives 115, no. 9 (September 2007): 1264–70, doi:10.1289/ehp.9951; Rudolf Jaenisch and Adrian Bird, "Epigenetic Regulation of Gene Expression: How the Genome Integrates Intrinsic and Environmental Signals," *Nature Genetics* 33 (2003): 245–54, doi:10.1038/ng1089.

12   Bruce H. Lipton, PhD, *The Biology of Belief: Unleashing the Power of Consciousness, Matter, & Miracles*, rev. ed. (Carlsbad, CA: Hay House, 2008).

13   Frank W. Booth, et al., "Waging War on Physical Inactivity: Using Modern Molecular Ammunition against an Ancient Enemy," *Journal of Applied Physiology* 93, no.1 (2002): 3–30, doi:10.1152.

14   S. Boyd Eaton, MD, and Melvin Konner, PhD, "Paleolithic Nutrition: A Consideration of Its Nature and Current Implications," *New England Journal of Medicine* 312, no. 5 (January 31, 1985): 283–9; Hussam Abuissa and James H. O'Keefe Jr., "Realigning Our 21st Century Diet and Lifestyle with Our Hunter-Gatherer Genetic Identity," *Directions in Psychiatry* 25 (2005): SR1–SR10; Janette B. Miller, Neil Mann, and Loren Cordain, "Paleolithic Nutrition: What Did Our Ancestors Eat?" in *Genes to Galaxies*, ed. Adam Selinger and Anne Green (Sydney, University of Sydney, 2009): 28–42; Pedro Carrera-Bastos, et al., "The Western Diet and Lifestyle and Diseases of Civilization," *Dovepress* 2011, no. 2 (March 2011): 15–35.

15   S. Boyd Eaton, MD, and Melvin Konner, PhD, "Paleolithic Nutrition: A Consideration of Its Nature and Current Implications," *The New England Journal of Medicine* 312, no. 5 (January 31, 1985): 283–9; Hussam Abuissa and James H. O'Keefe, Jr., "Realigning Our 21st Century Diet and Lifestyle with Our Hunter-Gatherer Genetic Identity," *Directions in Psychiatry* 25 (2005): SR1–SR10; Janette B. Miller, Neil Mann, and Loren Cordain, "Paleolithic Nutrition: What Did Our Ancestors Eat?" in *Genes to Galaxies*, ed. Adam Selinger and Anne Green (Sydney, University of Sydney, 2009): 28–42.

16   Quiping Gu, MD, et al., "Prescription Drug Use Continues to Increase: US Prescription Drug Data for 2007–2008," *NCHS Data Brief* 42.

17   Robert Preidt, "Prescription Drug Spending Doubled in Less Than a Decade," *USA Today* (September 4, 2010).

18   Ray Moynihan and Alan Cassels, *Selling Sickness: How the World's Biggest Pharmaceutical Companies are Turning Us All Into Patients* (New York: Nation Books, 2005).

19   Anne B. Martin, et al., "Growth In US Health Spending Remained Slow in 2010: Health Share of Gross Domestic Product Was Unchanged from 2009," *Health Affairs* 31, no. 1 (January 2012): 209, doi:10.1377/hlthaff.2011.1135.

20   International Communications Research for the American Society of

Health-System Pharmacists, "Medication Use Among Older Americans" (Bethesda, MD: American Society of Health-System Pharmacists, 2001), http://www.ashp.org/s_ashp/docs/files/PR_Over65.pdf.

21   S. Wu and A. Green, "Projection of Chronic Illness Prevalence and Cost Inflation" (Santa Monica, CA.: RAND Health, October 2000); V. M. Freid, A. B. Bernstein, M. A. Bush, "Multiple Chronic Conditions among Adults Aged 45 and Over: Trends Over the Past 10 Years," NCHS Data Brief 100 (Hyattsville, MD: National Center for Health Statistics, 2012).

22   Hussam Abuissa and James H. O'Keefe Jr., "Realigning Our 21st Century Diet and Lifestyle With Our Hunter-Gatherer Genetic Identity," *Directions in Psychiatry* 25 (2005): SR1–SR10.

23   M. Shields, M. D. Carroll, and C. L. Ogden, "Adult Obesity Prevalence in Canada and the United States," NCHS Data Brief 56 (Hyattsville, MD: National Center for Health Statistics, 2011); Cynthia L. Ogden, PhD, et al., "Prevalence of Obesity in the United States, 2009–2010," NCHS Data Brief 82 (Hyattsville, MD: National Center for Health Statistics, 2012); Cheryl D. Fryar, MSPH, Margaret D. Carroll, MSPH, and Cynthia L. Ogden, PhD, "Prevalence of Overweight, Obesity, and Extreme Obesity Among Adults: United States, Trends 1960–1962 through 2009–2010" (Hyattsville, MD: National Center for Health Statistics, 2012), http://www.cdc.gov/nchs/data/hestat/obesity_adult_09_10/obesity_adult_09_10.pdf.

24   Cynthia L. Ogden, PhD, et al., "Prevalence of Obesity in the United States, 2009–2010," NCHS Data Brief 82 (Hyattsville, MD: National Center for Health Statistics, 2012); K. M. Flegal, et al., "Prevalence and Trends in Obesity among US Adults, 1999–2000," *Journal of the American Medical Association* 288, no. 14 (2002): 1723–27; Ogden CL, Flegal KM, Carroll MD, Johnson CL, "Prevalence and Trends in Overweight among US Children and Adolescents, 1999–2000," *Journal of the American Medical Association* 288, no. 14 (2002): 1728–32.

25   World Health Organization, "The World Health Report 2000: Health Systems Improving Performance" (Geneva: World Health Organization, 2000), http://www.who.int/whr/2000/en/whr00_en.pdf.

26   Frank W. Booth, et al., "Waging War on Physical Inactivity: Using Modern Molecular Ammunition against an Ancient Enemy," *Journal of Applied Physiology* 93, no.1 (2002): 3–30, doi:10.1152.

27   American Cancer Society, "Cancer Facts & Figures 2010" (Atlanta: American Cancer Society, 2010), http://www.cancer.org/acs/groups/content/@nho/documents/document/acspc-024113.pdf.

28   American Diabetes Association, "Economic Costs of Diabetes in the US in

2012," *Diabetes Care* (2013) DOI:10.2337/dc12-2625.

29   E. A. Finkelstein, et al., "Annual Medical Spending Attributable to Obe-
     sity: Payer- and Service-Specific Estimates," *Health Affairs* 28, no. 5 (2009):
     w822–w831.

30   J. E. Everhart, ed., "The Burden of Digestive Diseases in the United States,"
     NIH Publication No. 09-6443 (Washington, DC: US Government Printing
     Office, 2008).

31   E. Yelin, et al., "National and State Medical Expenditures and Lost Earnings
     Attributable to Arthritis and Other Rheumatic Conditions—United States,
     2003," *Morbidity and Mortality Weekly Report* 56, no. 1 (2007): 4–7.

32   Ethel S. Siris, MD, et al., "Identification and Fracture Outcomes of Undiag-
     nosed Low Bone Mineral Density in Postmenopausal Women. Results From
     the National Osteoporosis Risk Assessment," *Journal of the American Medical
     Association* 286 (2001): 2815–22, doi:10.1001/jama.286.22.2815.

33   F.M. Scherer, "The Link Between Gross Profitability and Pharmaceutical
     R&D Spending," *Health Affairs* 20, no. 5 (September/October 2001): 216–20;
     National Science Foundation table H-3, "Company and Other (Except Fed-
     eral) Funds for Industrial R&D Performance, by Industry and by Size of Com-
     pany: 1953–98" and "Technical Notes for 1998," available at http://www.nsf.
     gov/statistics/iris/search_hist.cfm?indx=10.

34   Qiuping Gu, MD, PhD, Charles F. Dillon, MD, PhD, and Vicki L. Burt, ScM,
     RN, "Prescription Drug Use Continues to Increase: U.S. Prescription Drug
     Data for 2007–2008," *NCHS Data Brief* 42 (September 2010), http://www.
     cdc.gov/nchs/data/databriefs/db42.htm.

35   Gary Null, PhD, et al., "Death By Medicine," *Life Extension Magazine* (March
     2004).

36   K. J. Karren, et al., *Mind Body Health* (San Francisco: Benjamin Cummings,
     2010), 28; Walter Bradford Cannon, *Bodily Changes in Pain, Hunger, Fear and
     Rage: An Account of Recent Researches into the Function of Emotional Excite-
     ment* (New York: D. Appleton & Co., 1915); S. A. McLeod, "What is the Stress
     Response" (2010), http://www.simplypsychology.org/stress-biology.html.

37   Dr. James L. Chestnut was one of the first to bring this point to my attention.
     His work has been greatly influential in my thinking. Chestnut holds a bachelor
     of physical education degree and a master of science degree in exercise physiol-
     ogy with a specialization in neurological adaptation, he is a doctor of chiroprac-
     tic, and holds a post-graduate certification in wellness lifestyle. Dr. Chestnut is
     also the author of *The Wellness and Prevention Paradigm* (TWP Press, 2011).

38 Gail King, "Type II Diabetes, the Modern Epidemic of American Indians in the United States," Indian Health Service Division of Diabetes Treatment and Prevention (June 2012), http://anthropology.ua.edu/bindon/ant570/Papers/King/king.htm.

39 Marcus J. Hamilton, et al., "Nonlinear Scaling of Space Use in Human Hunter-Gatherers," *Proceedings of the National Academy of Sciences 11,* no. 104 (2007): 4765–69, DOI: 10.1073/pnas.0611197104; F. L. Dunn, "Epidemiological Factors: Health and Disease in Hunter-Gatherers" in *Man the Hunter,* eds. R. B. Lee and I. DeVore I (Chicago: Aldine Publishing, 1968), 221–28; P. Moodie, "Australian Aborigines" in *Western Diseases: Their Emergence and Prevention*, eds. H. C. Trowell and D. P. Burkitt (Cambridge, MA: Harvard University Press, 1981), 154–67.

40 Michael Gurven and Hillard Kaplan, "Longevity among Hunter-Gatherers: A Cross-Cultural Examination," *Population and Development Review* 33, no. 2 (2007): 321–65.

41 F. W. Booth, et al., "Waging War on Physical Inactivity: Using Modern Molecular Ammunition against An Ancient Enemy," *Journal of Applied Physiology* 93 (2002): 3–30.

42 Ibid.; Boyd Eaton & Stanley Eaton, "An Evolutionary Perspective on Human Physical Activity: Implications for Health," *Comparative Biochemistry and Physiology Part A, Molecular and Integrative Technology* 136 (2003): 153–59; C. K. Roberts and J. B. Barnard, "Effects of Exercise and Diet on Chronic Disease," *Journal of Applied Physiology* 98 (2005): 3–30; J. Schmahmann, "From Movement to Thought: Anatomic Substrate of the Cerebellar Contribution to Cognitive Processing," *Human Brain Mapping* 4 no. 3 (1996): 174–98, doi: 10.1002/(SICI)1097-0193(1996)4:3<174::AID-HBM3>3.0.CO;2-0; Eric P. Jensen, *Learning with the Body In Mind* (San Diego: The Brain Store, 2000).

43 D. W. Dunstan, et al., "Associations of TV Viewing and Physical Activity with the Metabolic Syndrome in Australian Adults," *Diabetologia* 48 (2005): 2254–61; F. B. Hu, et al., "Television Watching and Other Sedentary Behaviors In Relation to Risk of Obesity and Type 2 Diabetes Mellitus In Women," *Journal of the American Medical Association* 289 (2003): 1785–91; P. T. Katzmarzyk, et al. "Sitting Time and Mortality From All Causes, Cardiovascular Disease, and Cancer," *Medicine and Science in Sports Exercise* 41 (2009): 998–1005.

44 "Prevalence of Physical Activity, Including Lifestyle Activities Among Adults—United States, 2000–2001," *Morbidity and Mortality Weekly Report* 52 no. 32 (August 15, 2003): 764–69; James M. Rippe, MD, Theodore J.

Angelopoulos, PhD, MPH, and William Rippe, MD, "Lifestyle Medicine and Health Care Reform," *American Journal of Lifestyle Medicine* 3 (2009): 421–24; H. Abuissa, J. H. O'Keefe, and L. Cordain, "Realigning Our 21st Century Diet and Lifestyle With Our Hunter-Gatherer Genetic Identity," *Directions in Psychiatry* 25 (2005): SR1–SR10.

45   Boyd Eaton & Stanley Eaton, "An Evolutionary Perspective on Human Physical Activity: Implications for Health," *Comparative Biochemistry and Physiology Part A, Molecular and Integrative Technology* 136 (2003): 153–59; L. Cordain, R. W. Gotshall, and S. B. Eaton III, "Physical Activity, Energy Expenditure and Fitness: An Evolutionary Perspective," *International Journal of Sports Medicine* 19 no. 5 (1998): 328–35.

46   Dr. Lynn Becker, "The Feeding Mistake Linked to the Cause of Most Disease—Are You Making It?" http://healthypets.mercola.com/sites/healthypets/archive/2013/04/01/raw-food-diet-part-1.aspx.

47   Boyd S. Eaton, MD, and M. Konner, PhD, "Paleolithic Nutrition: A Consideration of Its Nature and Current Implications," *New England Journal of Medicine* 312 (1985): 283–89.

48   Ibid.; S. B. Eaton, S. B. Eaton III, and M. Konner, "Paleolithic Nurtrition Revisited: A Twelve Year Retrospective on its Nature and Implications," *European Journal of Clinical Nutrition* 51 (1997): 207–16; H. Abuissa, J. H. O'Keefe, and L. Cordain, "Realigning Our 21st Century Diet and Lifestyle with Our Hunter-Gatherer Genetic Identity," *Directions in Psychiatry* 25 (2005): SR1–SR10; J. Brand-Miller, N. Mann, L. Cordain, "Paleolithic Nutrition: What Did Our Ancestors Eat?" in *Genes to Galaxies*, eds. A. Selinger and A. Green (Sydney: University of Sydney, 2009), 28–42; P. Carrera-Bastos, et al., "The Western Diet and Lifestyle and Diseases of Civilization," *Journal of Research Reports in Clinical Cardiology* 2 (2011): 215–35.

49   Michael Gurven and Hillard Kaplan, "Longevity among Hunter-Gatherers: A Cross-Cultural Examination," *Population and Development Review* 33, no. 2 (2007): 321–65.

50   "Follow the Water, Finding A Perfect Match For Life," NASA Fact Sheet: FS-2006-10-131-LaRC (April 16, 2007): http://www.nasa.gov/vision/earth/everydaylife/jamestown-water-fs.html.

51   C.L. Chen, et al., "A Mechanism by which Dietary Trans Fats Cause Atherosclerosis," *Journal of Nutritional Biochemistry* 22, no. 7 (2011): 649–55, doi: 10.1016/j.jnutbio.2010.05.004; J. M. Smith, *Genetic Roulette: The Documented Health Risks of Genetically Engineered Foods* (Fairfield, IA: Yes! Books, 2007), 130; A. Pusztai, *Genetically Modified Foods: Are They a Risk to Human/*

Animal Health? http://www.actionbioscience.org/biotechnology/pusztai. html (2001); Catherine Paddock, "High-Fructose Corn Syrup Fuelling Type 2 Diabetes Epidemic," Medical News Today (Dec. 2, 2012), http://www. medicalnewstoday.com/articles/ 253484.php; John S. White, "Straight Talk about High-Fructose Corn Syrup: What It Is and What It Ain't," *American Journal of Clinical Nutrition* 88, no. 6 (2008): 716S–21S; M. D. Schorin, "High-Fructose Corn Syrups, Part 1: Composition, Consumption and Metabolism," *Nutrition Today* 40 (2005): 248–52; T. J. Maher and R. J. Wurtman, "Possible Neurologic Effects of Aspartame, A Widely Used Food Additive," *Environmental Health Perspectives* 75 (1987): 53; M. Soffritti, et al., "Lifespan Exposure to Low Doses of Aspartame Beginning During Prenatal Life Increases Cancer Effects in Rats," *Environmental Health Perspectives* 115, no. 9 (2007): 1293; R. Walker and J. R. Lupien, "The Safety Evaluation of Monosodium Glutamate," *Journal of Nutrition* 130, no. 4 (2000), 1049S–52S; K. Oh, et al., "Dietary Fat Intake and Risk of Coronary Heart Disease in Women: 20 Years of Follow-up of the Nurses' Health Study," *American Journal of Epidemiology* 161, no. 7 (2005), 672–79.

52   T. H. Holmes and R. H. Rabe, "The Social Readjustment Rating Scale," *Journal of Psychosomatic Research* 11 (1967), 213–18.

53   P. Carrera-Bastos, et al., "The Western Diet and Lifestyle and Diseases of Civilization," *Journal of Research Reports in Clinical Cardiology* 2 (2011): 215–35.

54   Stephen R. Covey, *The 7 Habits of Highly Effective People: Restoring the Character Ethic* (New York: Free Press, 2004).

55   M.D. Anway, et al., "Epigenetic Transgenerational Actions of Endocrine Disrupters and Male Fertility," *Science* 308 (2005): 1466–469; David Crews, et al., "Transgenerational Epigenetic Imprints on Mate Preference," *Proceedings of the National Academy of Sciences* 104, no. 14 (2007): 5942–946.

56   Andrea Lu, "Study: Food Additive Limits Longevity," *The Daily Californian*, February 8, 2006: http://archive.dailycal.org/article.php?id=23616.

57   Nancy Nelson, "The Majority of Cancers Are Linked to the Environment," *Benchmarks* 4, no. 3 (2004): 1.

58   Joyce M. Lee, et al., "Getting Heavier, Younger: Trajectories of Obesity Over the Life Course," *International Journal of Obesity* 34, no. 4 (2010): 614–23, doi: 10.1038/ijo.2009.235.

INDEX

V

W

Y

ABOUT THE AUTHOR

Using a hands-on approach, Dr. Jason Sonners, DC, DIBAK, DCBCN, CCWP, evaluates the structural, bio-chemical, and emotional causes of disease. By looking at the body holistically and addressing lifestyle habits and tendencies, Dr. Sonners helps his patients realize and express their body's full health potential.

Sonners graduated summa cum laude from New York Chiropractic College (NYCC). While attending NYCC, he received extensive training in Active Release Technique, Applied Kinesiology, exercise rehabilitation, nutrition, and injury prevention. Sonners has a B.S. in Exercise Physiology from Ithaca College.

Always striving to integrate new knowledge and practical experience, Sonners has earned his Diplomate of the Chiropractic Board of Clinical Nutrition (DCBCN) and the Diplomate of the International Board of Applied Kinesiology (DIBAK). He combines his knowledge and experience in chiropractic, exercise, and nutrition to provide unique treatment protocols to help and heal patients regardless of their health and fitness backgrounds.